SILVER
LININGS

SILVER LININGS

TRIUMPHS OF THE CHRONICALLY ILL AND PHYSICALLY CHALLENGED

Edited by

SHAENA ENGLE

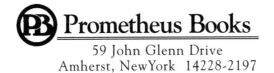 **Prometheus Books**

59 John Glenn Drive
Amherst, New York 14228-2197

Published 1997 by Prometheus Books

01 00 99 98 97   5 4 3 2 1

Library of Congress Cataloging-in-Publication Data

Silver linings : triumphs of the chronically ill and physically challenged /
    edited by Shaena Engle.
        p.   cm.
    Includes bibliographical references.
    ISBN 1–57392–171–8 (cloth : alk. paper)
    1. Chronically ill—Biography. 2. Physically handicapped—
Biography. I. Engle, Shaena.
RC108.S54   1997
362.1′092′2—dc21
[B]   97–37778
                                                                           CIP

Printed in the United States of America on acid-free paper

For Mary Jiry and Anne Engle,
my grandmother and mother,
who always take care of me when I am sick.

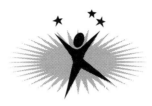

Contents

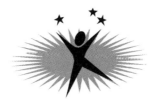

Acknowledgments

I am grateful to many people who helped my vision become a book. Without their dedication, support, and encouragement this project would not have been possible:

All of the contributors who took the time and effort to participate in this book, as well as their many projects providing education, inspiration, and funding to help thousands of people worldwide.

Alan Kellock, my agent, who believed in and devoted countless hours to this project from the beginning.

Kathy Deyell and Steven L. Mitchell at Prometheus, for editing and publishing my dream.

Anne, Ray, and Elysa Engle, my mother, father, and sister, who take care of me when I am sick. They also provided support, guidance, and encouragement during the four years that I worked on *Silver Linings*.

Joyce Curran taught me to always have confidence and strive for my goals. She was a wonderful teacher and her lessons have helped me throughout my life. Leeza Hoyt served as my professional mentor. She taught me the foundation for being a successful publicist and always provides guidance and support. Thanks to Mary Boston, Tammy Rivera, Al Schwartz, and Nuria Jenkins for also providing direction.

Carol Ross and Lyle McEachin, two special people, for their friendship and many hours listening to ideas and offering suggestions.

Alan Weinberger and Arthur Waltuch, my rheumatologists, who make time to see me and help me heal. Also, my nutritionist, Linda Sherman, for keeping me fit.

Lauren Arnold and Scott Ceiner, who shared my childhood and still make me smile today.

Don Hartley and Paul Bishop, both exceptional lawyers, for sharing their knowledge and experience so freely.

Darin Kinoshita, Sachi Okomoto, Pam Gallo, Grahm Martin, Susie and Gus Marino, Debbie Tierney, Shelley Cockrell, Michael Gurrieri, Cindy Quan, Roger Downing, Trisha Spellman, Nicole Rosencrantz, Steve Aboud, Anthony Robbins, the Tintocalis, Meislin, and Dullabaun families, Otis and Bill Jiry, Lee Shalom, Bob Davis, Grace Ho, and everyone at Enlace for their constant friendship and support.

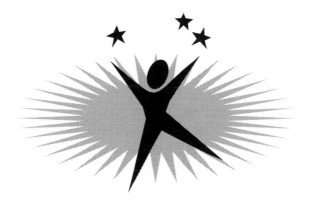

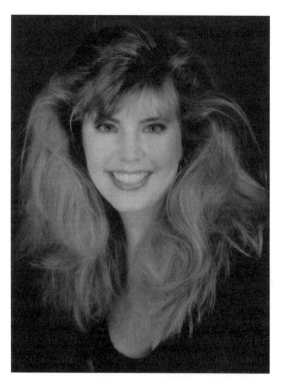

Shaena Engle

Shaena Engle was diagnosed with systemic lupus erythe-matosus at the age of sixteen. She has since met and talked with many other people who suffer from a variety of chronic illnesses and over the years she has been struck by how many of them seem to develop a greater understanding of and appreciation for life from the experience of coming to terms with their own affliction. She compiled the book Silver Linings *to share some of these stories. Ms. Engle heads a successful marketing consulting firm in Los Angeles and is currently working on her next book. A portion of her proceeds from this book will be donated to Athletes and Entertainers for Kids, a Los Angeles–based charity that helps enrich the lives of children diagnosed with chronic illnesses.*

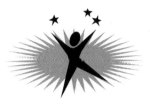

Introduction

The idea behind *Silver Linings* originated fifteen years ago. At the age of sixteen, I was diagnosed with systemic lupus erythematosus (SLE), a disease that I could barely pronounce and knew nothing about. It took a six-month period and many visits to different specialists to correctly diagnose my condition, which I share with an estimated 500,000 people in the United States, 80 percent of whom are women. Normally the immune system produces proteins, called antibodies, that fight bacteria, viruses, and germs. In people who have lupus, a malfunction occurs in some of the cells of the immune system. An increased number of antibodies are created and begin attacking normal, healthy tissue. In other words, the body begins attacking itself. Many people with lupus have high amounts of these self-fighting antibodies, therefore lupus is considered an "autoimmune" disease. Instead of fighting off infection, my antibodies attacked healthy tissue and destroyed my kidneys, although any or all of my organs could become targets. When foreign cells (viruses, bacteria, or germs) invade my body, my immune system malfunctions and overproduces antibodies to fight the invading cells, causing inflammation. I suffered from a rash on my face, across the bridge of my nose and my upper cheeks, resembling a "butterfly" pattern; oral ulcers; arthritis; kidney disease; hair loss; mood swings; constant fatigue; and low-grade fevers.

During the first year of my illness I was very sick. There were times when I thought that I was dying. I was tired of taking medication, getting blood tests, and always feeling fatigued. I felt confused, helpless, and unmotivated. I received lots of advice from doctors, family members, and friends, little of which was helpful although it was heartfelt. What I needed was guidance from those who had gone through similar situations who could offer advice on how to live with a chronic illness and inspire me to keep on living, reconstruct my life, and set meaningful goals, which I felt I needed to keep me motivated to fight the disease and survive. I wrote a list of all the things that I would accomplish when I became well. One of the items on my list was to help others who shared my feelings of loneliness, confusion, and isolation.

My road to wellness was a long, hard journey. Through exercise, persistence, and humor I was able to stop taking prescribed immunosuppressants and steroids ten years after I became ill. I consider the day I stopped taking medication as the day I achieved the ability to function as a "normal" person again. I began working toward the goals that I had set for myself a decade previously.

I decided that a book sharing what others have learned from their experiences with serious chronic illness and loss would provide inspiration, hope, and guidance. Above all, I wanted to include stories of people who, despite their own physical circumstances and challenges, have made extraordinary contributions to society. I felt that those who had life-threatening illnesses and major health challenges which drastically changed their lives, inspiring them to plan better and work harder to achieve their goals and dreams than do most people who do not face such adversities, would provide inspiration not only to those who share similar situations, but to all who heard or read about their unique lives.

Each of the following stories focuses on how individuals found the strength to live fulfilling lives despite their circumstances. They reveal how their own battles with chronic illness and disabilities motivated them to help others and share what they have been able to accomplish as a consequence. These are stories of people whose experience with adversity not only altered their lives forever, it enriched them as well.

Living with lupus, I know firsthand what it's like to experience serious chronic illness. Coping with my illness forced me to discover my strengths and reconstruct my life, and I've emerged with both a deeper understanding of what I value in life and a fierce determination to achieve my dreams. My goal for this book is to help readers along a similar road to self-fulfillment.

Unchain Your Dreams

Raun Kaufman

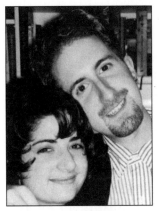

Raun Kaufman was diagnosed as autistic and retarded, with an IQ under 30, at the age of eighteen months. Undaunted, his parents, Barry and Samahria Kaufman, created a unique intervention program that completely cured Raun. His remarkable story is recounted in the best-selling book Son-Rise: The Miracle Continues *and in the NBC-TV movie* Son-Rise: A Miracle of Love. People *magazine,* Family Circle, Abnormal Psychology, *and other major publications have detailed Raun's journey out of autism. Raun went on to earn a degree in biomedical ethics from a leading Ivy League university. As a speaker at colleges and universities, Raun inspires students to work with developmentally challenged children in the daring way his parents once worked with him. The pioneering program responsible for his emergence from autism has grown into The Son-Rise Program® at The Option Institute, which now helps thousands of families around the world to "reach" their "unreachable" special needs children.*

When I am asked to speak about my experience with autism, it occurs to me that many people unconnected to this subject might see it as somewhat narrow in scope and probably irrelevant in their own lives. In fact, the case is precisely the oppo-

17

site. To illustrate this, I would like to not only tell my story, but to explain some of its underlying ideas. I strongly believe that the core behind the story is so relevant and so important that your adoption or even consideration of it can profoundly change your life and the lives of every single person that you touch.

Before my first birthday (in 1976), I had begun to withdraw from human contact. I would not look at people. When picked up and held, I would let my arms dangle lifelessly at my sides. Never did I make any attempt to speak, nor did I cry, yell, point, or do anything at all to communicate my wishes. Additionally, I began to exhibit unusual behaviors. I spent endless hours rocking back and forth, spinning plates, flapping my hands in front of my face, and staring into space.

As weeks turned to months, my parents grew increasingly more concerned about my condition. Having already had two daughters, they were familiar with the many phases children go through. Because my development was dramatically different from that of my sisters, my parents took me to a number of specialists to find out what was happening to me and what they could do about it. They wanted answers, suggestions, insights, and, above all, some direction—a trail to set their feet upon.

However, events began to spiral in a direction that was neither heartening nor empowering. First came whole batteries of tests. Then the shaking heads. After that, the labels, spoken with the finality of a death sentence. Then more tests. Shaking heads. Tapping pencils. More labels. Finally, the diagnosis: a classic case of infantile autism. Profound retardation. A tested IQ of below 30. Possible deafness. The prognosis, according to the specialists, was certain. Autism, considered by the medical community to be a severely incapacitating, life-long disability, was one of the truly irreversible, incurable, and unfathomable afflictions of the world, and there was nothing—absolutely nothing—that my parents could do about it. My parents were informed that autism is a neurological disorder that typically appears during the first three years of life and is characterized by extreme lack of eye contact, repetitious behavior such as flapping or rocking, withdrawal from people, and an inability to show emotion, communicate, or process information. I would never learn to speak, read, or play baseball. I would never drive a car, write a poem, hang out with friends, or go out on a date. I would, in fact, never learn to communicate in any meaningful way. Like other autistic people, I would literally be "in my own world." I might, one day, after a great deal of therapy, learn to use silverware or maybe even to dress myself. Beyond that, my condition was hopeless. The best thing to do at this point was to put me in an institution where I could be properly "managed."

Clearly, this was not the inspiration my parents sought. Instead of empowerment, they were shown impotence. Rather than finding out what they could do, my parents were told what they could not do. If they truly wanted a path upon which to set their feet, they were going to have to carve one out of the wilderness themselves. And, wouldn't you know it, that is exactly what they did.

Turning their backs on the pessimism, rigidity, and hopelessness of the professionals, my parents decided to act on their own. What made their actions so groundbreaking was their perspective—one which went against the grain of everything that society teaches us about illness, challenges, love, and life itself. My parents looked at me and saw possibilities, not deficiencies.

They felt wonder, not horror. They looked at me, spinning in circles, flapping my hands, and saw an amazing little boy touching the sky in a world of his own creation.

People with the best of intentions, wishing to console my parents, said things like, "Oh, I'm so sorry," "What a tragedy," and "How awful for you." My parents knew, however, that they never wanted to see me as tragic or awful in any way. They could see the beauty in my condition, and they chose to embrace it.

From this radically different perspective grew the home-based, child-centered program that my parents developed for me. The core of the program was a totally nonjudgmental, accepting, and loving attitude. What does this mean in practice? First of all, it means that my parents did not see my autism as bad and never viewed any of my admittedly unusual behaviors as wrong or weird. They always totally accepted me exactly the way I was, whether I improved dramatically or remained completely unchanged. And foremost, they loved me completely and unconditionally, regardless of whether or not that love was returned.

For three and a half years my parents worked with me, twelve hours a day, seven days a week. Unlike the professionals, whose goal with special children is to eliminate "bad" behaviors and teach "good" ones in an effort to make the children "normal," my mother and father sought connection above all. They wanted to reach out to me and build a bridge from their world to mine, a bridge they knew I would cross only by choice—never by coercion.

Aside from being much more humane and respectful than "traditional" treatments, there is also an inherent logic in this approach. Let's take, for example, the approach that the professionals offered my parents. Children treated under the "standard" system are physically manipulated against their will, and punished when they do not follow a prescribed regimen. Why on earth would autistic children have even the slightest desire to join a world that is the exact opposite of what they, or any of us, would want? These kids are shown a world marked by disapproval, physical force, condescension, and a total lack of control over their environment. Who would want that? Who would, after seeing such a world, do anything other than run away or push against it? I, for one, would catch the first flight out of there.

Imagine, on the other hand, that you are presented with a world where your every move was praised, where you were loved and supported no matter what, yet still always encouraged to do more, and where your wishes were respected wherever possible. Who wouldn't put in some serious overtime to reach that destination?

In truth, the program my parents created is based on the kind of love everyone wants but rarely, if ever, gets. Picture someone—a friend, a lover, a parent—loving you unconditionally and not judging you ever. What would that feel like? There isn't a person on the planet who doesn't dream of being loved this way. An autistic child could never receive a greater gift.

It is critical to understand that my parents were totally alone in their ideas and efforts. They had no cheering section. Their friends and family, by and large, deserted them outright or were completely unsupportive. Moreover, the doctors were vehemently opposed to everything my parents believed and were trying to accomplish. In my opinion, these factors make what my parents did even more astounding. It takes a lot of vision and guts to persevere when no one is on your side.

Most people believe that feeling sad and calling a situation horrible are the ways that we show how much we care. If we care about or love someone, the common belief is that we should try to "feel their pain," and commiserate with them about the awfulness of a given situation. The irony is that all of the "caring" that the people around my parents lavished upon them ultimately did me and my parents absolutely no good. It generated nothing but misery and impotence. Conversely, my parents, who cared for and loved me a great deal, *showed* that caring, not with sorrow and pessimism, but with excitement and optimism. This empowered them to act instead of talk, and to face their challenge instead of turning away.

My parents originally began working with me in the living room, but there were too many distractions. They needed a place where they could work with me uninterrupted for hours. They racked their brains in an effort to come up with the ideal place. It had to be away from the action, not too large, conducive to concentration, and, certainly, a very special place worthy of the momentous work ahead. Where, though, could such a place be? The answer came, clear as day: the bathroom. Yes, the bathroom. This incredible act of love and transformation took place somewhere between the sink and the toilet. But who was I to be picky?

When they first began their program with me, my parents did not have everything planned out in precise detail. Although they knew exactly the approach they wanted to take, they were not always 100 percent sure what course of action their approach dictated. To some degree, they made discoveries and breakthroughs as they went along.

One very important activity my parents did with me was to join me in whatever I was doing. If I was spinning a plate, they would get plates of their own and spin with me for hours. When I rocked, they would rock with me. This practice drew a lot of outside criticism. Many professionals argued that this was the worst thing my mother and father could do because it only reinforced my autistic behaviors. However, those people did not understand my parents' point of view and, consequently, they viewed my parents' actions through the colored glass of their own philosophy. Again, my mother and father were seeking connection first and foremost. Constantly bombarding me with disapproval and demands was not the way to achieve this. Joining me in my world, showing me that what I was doing was okay, was the best way to forge the kind of connection they were looking for. In fact, their first breakthrough with me came from exactly this activity.

I began, for the very first time, to actually look at my parents and make eye contact, the fundamental foundation of any connection. As I changed and grew, they adjusted the program accordingly. In sharp contrast to the "traditional" approach, my mother and father let me be the teacher. They used me as their guide, adjusting the program to fit where I was, not where I supposedly should be.

My progress was marked by slow change sandwiched between huge leaps and breakthroughs. By the time I was four, I had gone from a mute, self-stimulating, "unreachable," "hopeless" little boy to an outgoing, verbal, fun-loving kid. The energy, dedication, love, daring, and relentless optimism that my parents displayed helped me to emerge completely from the shell of my autism without any trace of my former condition. The spectacular luck that I had to get the parents that I got quite honestly dumbfounds me. When I think about what could have been, I have to catch my breath.

What really makes my story so amazing and meaningful, in my opinion, is not so much the outcome (though, of course, I have no complaints about that) but the way my parents looked at and reacted to my autism. Though I am well aware of the fact that it is my dramatic recovery that captures people's imagination, there is so much more to see than that.

I am often asked what I have learned from my experience, and 90 percent of my answer has nothing to do with the end result. One key thing I learned is that the meaning of events in our lives is not contained within those events but in our reaction to them. My autism could have been just another sad, meaningless tragedy in the world. Do you know why it wasn't? Not because I got better, but because my parents gave it meaning long before I made any improvements. They faced something most people would see as unquestionably awful and tragic and decided to see it as the best thing that had ever happened—before they had any idea what the outcome would be. They saw the wonder in their situation, and, in so doing, they made it wondrous! They gave the event its greatness, not vice versa.

My story is not the tale of a family overcoming strife and hardship. My parents skipped over the whole strife bit. There was great challenge, but, for our family, there was no hardship. Rather, it is the story of people who took something others called ugly and made it beautiful. It is the story of a set of parents who, as my father wrote in his book *Son Rise: The Miracle Continues,** decided to "kiss the ground that the others had cursed."

What is vital to understand is that my parents were

---

*Barry Neil Kaufman, *Son Rise: The Miracle Continues* (Tiburon, Calif.: H. J. Kramer, 1994), p. 4.

not born with some special ability to give events greatness. We can all do this, and we can do it every single day! We can take anything that happens to us, whether others call it good or bad, and make it great by choosing to see it that way. We can get excited instead of discouraged, inspired instead of depressed. How different would our life experiences be if we decided to do this on a regular basis?

Another thing I've learned is to let those around you live their own lives, but don't let them live yours. Only you know what the right path for you is, although I'll be the first to admit that it doesn't always feel that way. Go your own way, do what feels right, and stick to your guns. If my parents had taken anyone's advice but their own, I'd be rotting in an institution right now.

I have a few words to say about hope. Many professionals argue against what my parents are teaching families (and what I am saying to you right now) on the grounds that it fosters false hope. This irritates me because putting the words "false" and "hope" together in the same sentence is like mixing ketchup and ice cream, it's a nasty tasting combination. These two words do not fit together. They are based on the idea that there are times when hoping can be false or incorrect. My entire life is a product of "false hope" and so are the lives of many others. Hope is the spark that ignites the human spirit and nothing can ever be bad or wrong about it. Not ever. In fact, hopelessness breeds inaction. Please do not listen to anyone who argues against hoping for things you want. Your hopes are better off *up* than they are *down*.

The last big thing I learned from my experience is to be unrealistic. I know this sounds a little nutty but I'll explain. All of the people around my parents—friends, doctors, family—kept telling them to "be realistic" about their situation and about me. However, any realistic person would have said, "The kid is autistic. He has an IQ of below 30. His condition is not curable. People do not recover from this kind of thing. There is plenty of evidence to prove just how unreachable he is—the doctors themselves showed it to me. Even if I had the time to set up and implement my own program for this boy, I have been given a million reasons why it wouldn't work, anyway. The best thing to do is to make sure he is properly taken care of and move on." This is, in fact, what thousands of compassionate, caring people say every day about thousands of autistic children.

My parents, on the other hand, were decidedly unrealistic in their dealings with me. They ignored the criticism, the scorn, and the mountain of evidence against the possibility of a recovery and tried to accomplish the impossible. Does this make them inherently superior to the "realists"? No. But look at what they were able to do when they unchained their dreams! If anything is possible, and I believe that it is, then why should anyone have to give up the opportunity to attempt something because someone else calls it "impossible"?

Think about it. Every great discovery and achievement in history was accomplished by unrealistic people. Martin Luther King Jr., Alexander Graham Bell, Susan B. Anthony—none of these people was realistic. End segregation? Make people's voices travel along a tiny wire? Women and men, equal? It sounds silly now, but before the deed was done, these people's ideas were ridiculed and labeled totally unrealistic. Now, however, they are fact.

I have to be honest. Being unrealistic isn't always my forté. I'm a pretty practical guy, and I often take the sensible route. Sometimes this means that I do not even bother attempting something because I think, "No way. There is no way that can be done. It's impossible. Unfortunately, this is precisely the type of thinking that could have landed me in an institution for my entire life. I can be sure that when I *do* think this way, everything will be nice and predictable. However, when I decide to forget the conventional wisdom, I can accomplish more and reach higher than I ever could have by being realistic. Without question, I, rather than my external situation, am my own biggest limiter. Being unrealistic doesn't guarantee me the result I want, but it opens up a lot of possibilities.

After my recovery, my father, who, in my humble opinion, is a phenomenal writer, wrote a book entitled *Son-Rise.** *Son-Rise* is a touching, inspiring account of my parents' experience with me. It also provides a detailed outline of the philosophy behind the program that my parents developed. This incredibly empowering philosophy, called the Option Process®, focuses on beliefs as the driving force of our emotions and actions and enables people to become happier and clearer by choice. Another one of my father's books, *Happiness Is a Choice,*† explains how to integrate this philosophy into your everyday life.

Although *Son-Rise* was written partly to share my parents' experience with other parents of special children so that they could find hope and possibly help their children, people from all walks of life picked up the book

*Barry Neil Kaufman, *Son-Rise* (New York; Harper & Row, 1976). This book, now out of print, has been replaced by the newly revised *Son-Rise: The Miracle Continues,* which will be discussed shortly.

*Barry Neil Kaufman, *Happiness Is a Choice* (New York: Fawcett Columbine, 1991).

and were deeply moved by it. Later, in 1979, NBC made the book into an award-winning, feature-length television movie called *Son Rise: A Miracle of Love* (my parents wrote the screenplay), which was viewed by millions of people across the globe.

People began to come to my parents, both to learn how to help their special children and to apply the Option Process® to their own lives. One of the first families to do this was the Sotos. The Sotos read *Son-Rise* and came from Mexico to ask my parents for help with their autistic son, Robertito. My parents volunteered to help the Sotos, and, for over a year, worked tirelessly with them. By the time the Sotos went back to Mexico, Robertito had come quite a long way from the lifeless, unresponsive child he had been when I first met him. The entire story is told in my father's book, *A Miracle to Believe In.** His parents, after working with my parents, were able to continue the program after they left.

Although I was only five years old at the time, I participated in this program while the Sotos were in the United States. I remember my involvement quite clearly, and I can tell you that, for me, working with Robertito was an extraordinary experience. Though I understood the tenets of my parents' program and philosophy, I also viewed the situation through very young eyes. This meant that I could work with Robertito, encouraging him, joining him in his behaviors, and still basically feel like I was playing with him, since he was a boy close to my age. I feel like this was an asset because I didn't carry around the baggage that an adult might have. For instance, I didn't judge myself or Robertito if

---

*Barry Neil Kaufman, *A Miracle to Believe In* (New York: Fawcett Crest, 1981, 1982).

he did not respond or "improve." I didn't feel uncomfortable with his very unusual behaviors. Plus, I never felt then (nor do I feel now) that Robertito's (or any child's) autism was in any way a negative condition or a situation from which he needed to be rescued. What I believe now is that autism is an unpleasant experience only when autistic children are pushed and pulled against their will the way they are so often in "treatment facilities." Other than that, I think autism is, in many ways, a wonderful state to be in, and I see autistic children as beautiful, special beings worthy of the utmost respect.

You may ask, then, why I would support efforts like those of my parents to help children move beyond their condition. My answer has two parts. The first is that I think our world (i.e., the world of "normal people") has much to offer, and I would want to give as many children possible a chance to get the most they could out of it. The second, and possibly more important, part of my answer is that we try to help children emerge from their autism more for ourselves than for them. We want to be able to interact and communicate with them. The only way that this can happen is if they emerge from autism, at least to some degree. I might add that I do not think there is anything to be ashamed of about this motive for helping children who are autistic. In the final analysis, they are the ones who will make the decision. All we can do is help give them the tools to make that choice. From there, ultimately, it is they who will move in one direction or another. Whatever direction they choose, I believe that children with autism can live happy and meaningful lives.

Let's move forward a few years. As more and more people started coming to my parents for help, they realized that the best thing to do to reach all of them was to come up with a place where families could come to learn how to start their own Son-Rise Program® and where individuals could learn in more detail about the Option Process®. Thus, in 1983, my parents founded The Option Institute and Fellowship in Sheffield, Massachusetts, a nonprofit learning center where families, groups, couples, and individuals come from across the country and around the world to learn how to live happier, healthier, and more productive lives. Some of these people are families with special children. Others are adults challenged by adversity—from cancer to divorce to the loss of a loved one. Still others are people who just want to live happier lives.

In 1994, my father wrote *Son-Rise: The Miracle Continues*. This book has a foreword, which I wrote, and three parts. The first is an expanded version of the original story. The second part follows my family and me over the past two decades, ending when I'm twenty years old. The third section tells the story of five families who came to The Option Institute, started their own Son-Rise Program®, and made incredible leaps with their special children.

Because of my parents' work, I have had the opportunity to talk with parents of special children from many different countries and throughout the United States. It is fascinating to me how much these families, with such diverse backgrounds, have in common. They want so much to help their children, and yet so many of them have had their hope vigorously stamped out by books, organizations, professionals, and sometimes even family and friends. I feel lucky to have been able to speak with and cheer on so many of these families. Also, when I hear about how special children are handled by professionals, I want to do something to change it.

Whenever I speak at a university or other similar arena, I always keep in mind that many of the people in the audience will be the professionals of the future. It is these people whom I want so badly to reach, so that, as time passes, more and more special children will be treated with the love and respect they deserve.

In all honesty, though, I must admit that I have some ambivalence about the position in which I find myself. I am still, even after all these years, somewhat taken aback by the intensity of the reaction that some parents have upon meeting me. People don't realize that it can feel strange to have something that has always been a given in my life, namely the fact that I am no longer autistic, evoke such emotion and inspiration for so many people. I sometimes feel caught between my desire to help people and my determination to live my life on my own terms, without being deprived of my privacy and without being judged, whether positively or negatively, because of my past.

Surprisingly, I have encountered situations where people who have never seen or met me (usually individuals representing established interests that are threatened by my parents' successful methods) make blatantly false statements about me and the events of my life;* (for example that I'm in an institution, that I have difficulty communicating with people, or that I never made it through college). In one instance a man who has never met me was sharing incorrect information in a letter about me on the internet. When I responded to him, he

---

*Although it might seem odd to have people you don't know discussing you, because of the publicity generated through my parents' program, the books, and the movie, my history has been a topic of conversation on television and radio talk shows and has appeared in various magazines, including *People* and *Family Circle*.

was completely flabbergasted. He said he had written because he didn't want parents to get "false hope" from my story. Instead of false hope (which I've made clear I don't believe exists) the information they received was just plain false!

I want to set the record straight. I have had, thus far, a great life. I grew up excelling in school and enjoying a busy social life (when I was younger, I used to boast about how I was the first kid in my class to have a coed party). I spent my final three years of high school attending a college prep school in my area. To this day, I still keep in touch with almost all of my friends from public school and prep school.

I applied to several Ivy League colleges, and when I was admitted to Brown University in Providence, Rhode Island, my first choice, I was beyond ecstatic. I had a total blast at college and spent my junior year as an exchange student at Stockholm University in Sweden. I also got to travel a lot that year, and, with my trusty Eurail pass in hand, I visited almost every country in Europe.

I graduated from Brown with a degree in biomedical ethics. Although you may not be familiar with this field, it is extremely fascinating. It combines the subjects of philosophy, biology, political science, and sociology. If you are familiar with the controversies surrounding Dr. Kevorkian and assisted suicide, test tube babies, genetic engineering of humans, the price of pharmaceutical drugs, living wills, the AIDS crisis, or even what I have written about the treatment of autistic children, then you have had exposure to the field of biomedical ethics.

Originally, when I entered college, I wanted to go into business as a profession. However, while at Brown I discovered two interests that I never knew I had. These discoveries quite literally altered the course of my life, both in the long and short term. The first interest I discovered was politics. I began to follow local and national elections very closely, to read and write about politically controversial issues, and to become involved in political groups on campus. During the 1992 election season, I spent a lot of time working on the campaign of one of the presidential candidates. Around this time I decided that, sometime down the road, I would run for national political office. I know the thought of Generation X taking hold of the reins of government strikes mortal fear into the hearts of some, but you can't fight the inevitable. I stumbled onto my second interest almost by accident. During my sophomore year in college, I saw a sign posted in one of the dorms about a summer enrichment program for kids called Exploration. This program, held on the campus of Wellesley College just outside of Boston, is world-renowned and teaches children from around the globe. The sign mentioned that Exploration was hiring residential advisors and teachers. So I applied and was interviewed.

Out of roughly seven hundred applicants from top universities and graduate schools across the nation, I was among sixty chosen to design and teach courses to junior high students at Exploration. I am thankful, in retrospect, that I was chosen. That summer was when I realized that teaching kids was one of my all-time favorite things to do in the world. I never would have known otherwise because I had absolutely no intention of ever entering the field of education. The whole experience turned my head around. I returned to Exploration each summer for the next three years, eventually receiving a promotion to help manage the program and supervise the staff.

After my last summer at Exploration, I began what

is widely considered the most dreaded stage of post-college life—a process known, in its abbreviated form, as: The What the Heck Are You Gonna Do with Your Life?/ Get a Clue/Quit Fooling Around/For Pete's Sake Choose Already/Above All Get Hired/Job and Career Search. Now, as most of you have probably read in newspaper and magazine articles, my entire generation is having collective heart palpitations over this process. I was no exception. I printed out enough variations of my résumé to wipe out a small rain forest. There were so many different things I wanted to do, I didn't know where to start. Because of my experience at Exploration, I knew that one of the areas in which I really wanted to work was education. However, I wanted business experience, too. How, though, would I ever find a job that combined these two disparate areas?

Lo and behold, I found just such a job. I interviewed at Score@Kaplan, a subsidiary of the *Washington Post* which operates innovative learning centers for kids around the country. Better still, they hired me. I am now one of the directors at a Score@Kaplan educational center in the Boston area. Incredibly, I get the best of both worlds. I get to work with kids of all ages on math, reading, writing, and spelling, and I get to handle the business side of the center as well. Also, Score@Kaplan has the same positive, enthusiastic, inventive approach to kids that I have, so it's a perfect fit.

I discovered something very interesting in the course of my career. When I'm with a young person, whether that child is one of the "normal" students I work with every day or one of the children with autism with whom I've worked in the past, I find that I am the very best of who I am. I am at my most dynamic, creative, and loving. Even if I am having an off day or I'm upset about something, I'm still at my best when I'm with kids. I have spoken with many other people who feel the same way. Even for those who do not, there is almost always some aspect of their life that is, for them, akin to my being with children. The question, then, is this: what would happen if we made our whole life a room full of kids? If I can shine when I'm with young people, why not put myself in that state of mind all day? Is such a thing possible? It's just some food for thought.

Needless to say, I get asked tons of questions by parents and others who meet me after reading the book or seeing the movie about my emergence from autism. There are, of course, some questions I get asked much more often than others. What am I like now? Do I get unhappy about things, or am I just incredibly together and content at all times? (Yes, I've actually been asked this question several times.) What kind of things do I like to do? Do my friends know about my past? If so, how do they react? What was it like growing up in my family? What are my plans for the future?

I will try to answer these questions as briefly as possible. First, in many ways, I'm a pretty regular guy. I work, I go out with my friends, I've had my share of girl-friends, I eat junk food, I go to the gym (these last two activities pretty much cancel each other out, unfortunately), I get sucked into bad TV shows, I get harassed by long distance telephone companies trying to get me to switch—you know, the basics. As you can probably tell from reading this essay, I try not to take myself or life in general too seriously.

Do I get ever get unhappy? Of course I do. There are plenty of times when I get upset or bummed out, but the difference for me is that I have no illusions about my un-happiness. I know that I can always choose to see a particular situation as either good or bad. Therefore, when I do get unhappy about something, I know that it is my decision to react that way, not the result of some outside event.

My interests vary widely. They include politics, political debate, medical issues, public speaking, and acting. Writing is a major hobby of mine as well. I've been working on a novel for ages, and one of these years, when I actually find myself with some free time, I will finish it and hopefully have it published. My favorite sports to play are tennis and volleyball. As far as my friends go, almost all of them know about my past. In the cases where people do not know, it is only because it hasn't come up, not because I have a problem with them knowing. The vast majority of my friends who do know my story don't really care, and that is exactly the way I like it.

Growing up in my family was terrific. I have been extraordinarily lucky to grow up in the family that I did, even aside from what my parents did when I was autistic. Throughout my childhood, my parents were extremely loving and supportive of me. I also had a very honest relationship with them, which I think is unusual. I did not have to hide things from my parents because they created an environment where it was safe to be honest. Did my parents ever do things that bugged me when I was a teenager? Sure, but they were so reasonable as parents that I didn't have a whole lot to rebel against while I was going through my teen years. Considering how most families operate, I sometimes have a hard time believing that I got such a lucky break with mine.

My plans for the future? I have several ideas, and I do not know as of yet which of them will come to pass, but here they are. I want to start an employment agency for the homeless, open a virtual reality movie theater, run a health-care consulting firm, help start a charter school (an experimental public school), develop a health care system that will cover all Americans, unite our tax and environmental policies into a cohesive system, develop a plan to reconnect the inner cities to the rest of America, and run for political office. Do you think all of these ambitions are unrealistic? You bet they are. I wouldn't have it any other way.

Being unrealistic, staying in touch with the very best of ourselves, loving someone without judgments or conditions, trusting ourselves, following our own compass, and hoping in the face of impossibility can change our lives in a big way, but it doesn't stop there. As we all know, these actions can alter the course of a child's life, a friend's life, and the life of anyone with whom we come into contact. Truly, we can use these visions to move mountains.

So the question still remains: If we can be unrealistic and we can bring beauty and meaning to the events in our lives and we can, in each and every moment, be loving and creative and passionate, and if we can take all of that and turn it loose upon the world, then what on earth are we waiting for? It is never too soon to quench our thirst for greatness.

For an information packet about the Option Institute and the Son-Rise Program®, please call 1(800)71–HAPPY [1(800)714–2779].

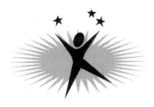

Laughter in the Dark

Alex Valdez

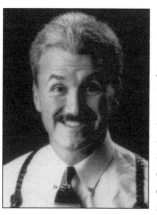

On June 6, 1977, Alex Valdez stepped onto the stage at the Comedy Store in Westwood, California, to become the first comedian with a disability. Born with congenital glaucoma, Alex has been totally blind since the age of seven. Over the last two decades he has appeared at comedy clubs and colleges across the country along with countless appearances on television and radio shows. Alex costarred on the award winning PBS documentary, "Look Who's Laughing" that showcased the talents and experiences of six comedians with disabilities. In the past few years Alex has expanded his career to include professional speaking, allowing him to share his message of courage to an even wider, more diverse audience.

In over two decades of performing nationally as a stand-up comedian, people are still amazed that I can laugh at being totally blind. I, on the other hand, have always been amazed how anyone could face the challenges we all have in our lives without a good sense of humor. I have found that laughter is one of the ultimate tools for keeping life's difficulties in proper perspective, and I have come to realize that my blindness has *not* been the greatest obstacle I have had to face in my life.

I was born the second child of Carmen and Alex Valdez in the city of Santa Ana, California. Until a routine visit to the pediatrician when I was six months old, my parents could not have been happier with our lives. Their first child was a girl and now they had a new son; a namesake for my father. We were the typical 1950s family until the visit to my pediatrician that changed my family's world. I was my parents' first full-term baby (my older sister had been born prematurely), and so any rate of development I had been making must have seemed normal. When the doctor voiced his concern about my vision, it came as a complete surprise to my parents. At the pediatrician's recommendation I was taken to an ophthalmologist for an evaluation of my eyesight.

My first visit to the specialist was a dismal failure. The doctor suspected that my vision problem might be glaucoma, and it was necessary to perform a test that would determine the pressure in my eyes to see if he was correct. All attempts to do so, however, were warded off by my thrashing and wailing. The decision was made to bring me back for a second attempt for an examination and this time they would put me under anesthesia for the test. In the 1950s, medicine had not yet abandoned the use of ether as a general anesthetic. Under the effects of the ether the doctor was able to take the eye pressure reading necessary to confirm the diagnosis of congenital glaucoma in my left eye. However, the ether proved to be too much for a nine-month-old baby and I went into respiratory arrest as my terrified father watched the doctor's frantic efforts to revive me. The doctor's resuscitation attempts were successful and I survived without any additional complications.

My family threw themselves into the battle to save my vision from the effects of the congenital glaucoma, a

rare condition that usually affects both eyes simultaneously. It is caused by a defect that obstructs the outward
flow of fluid from the eye, causing a chronic increase in
pressure. As the disease progresses, the optic nerve becomes damaged and blindness eventually occurs. Early
surgical treatment is the only real hope of preserving
any useful vision. My father put in long hours at work
to continue to support our family despite the mounting
doctor bills and the emotional pressures of having a sick
child. My grandmother, Mama Vicki, left the comfort of
her own home in Santa Barbara to live with us and provide care for my sister, Cathy, and physical and spiritual
support for my parents.

During these years my mother put all of her own
wants and needs aside, including a necessary surgery.
My mother was also disabled due to rheumatoid
arthritis, which is a form of arthritis that can affect
anyone, including children and the elderly, although the
disease usually begins in the young- to middle-adult
years. Over 2.5 million people in the world have rheumatoid arthritis, and women outnumber men by three
to one. The disease causes the white blood cells to move
from the bloodstream into the joint tissues, where the
joint fluid increases and the white cells produce antibodies and other substances that cause an overall sick
feeling. If the inflammation is chronic and does not respond well to treatment, destruction of cartilage, bone,
tendons, and ligaments can occur, leading to deformity
and possible permanent disability. The doctor gave my
mother the choice of controlling her condition by either
remaining in bed or taking a medication (cortisone) that
had questionable long-term side effects, including
bruising, thinning of the bones, and cataracts, to name
just a few. To allow her to care for her three young chil-

dren, which included taking me daily to the eye doctor, she chose the medication. The prolonged use of the cortisone eventually contributed to her becoming confined to a wheelchair, having her left leg amputated, and ultimately an early death from diabetes. Despite her own medical problems, she was always by my side. She agonized and prayed through the seven difficult surgeries the doctors performed on my eye. She comforted my screams as the pain of the surgeries and the glaucoma became overwhelming and when exhaustion from my thrashing finally overtook me, she lovingly held my hand every moment I slept.

During this time my family put all their energies into saving my vision. Each operation carried a risk for my life and each time my parents feared that I might not survive. My mother would quietly slip away to the hospital chapel during each surgery and pray that her child would come through another operation safely. Mama Vicki became the religious head of our family. Her deep faith gave my parents the spiritual lift that kept them going through those difficult years. It was Mama Vicki's vision that finally gave my mother peace. Before one of my many surgeries my grandmother had a vision and in it she saw me as an old man with grey hair. Everyone put a great deal of faith in Mama Vicki's visions and when she told my family of what she had seen, my mother's fear was replaced with a strong faith that I would survive and live to be an old man. Of course, little did anyone suspect at the time that the full head of grey hair Mama Vicki envisioned would arrive in my early thirties.

Dr. Peal was a wonderful, caring man who did everything that contemporary medical knowledge would allow. He generously opened his home nights, weekends, and holidays to provide care and comfort to me when the pain of my glaucoma did not conform to regular office hours. I remember in particular the Christmas Eve when I was three years old; the pain from the eye became so unbearable that on Christmas morning my parents packed me in the family car and took me to Dr. Peal's home. I have been fortunate in that time has allowed me to forget the pain I endured that night, but my sister has not allowed me to forget. Due to my screaming she woke just in time to see our Aunt Rita filling the Christmas stockings with fruit. Because of me, at the age of five she was robbed forever of her childhood belief in Santa.

As kind as my doctors were, the medical profession had not yet taken time to address the psychological needs of children as patients. The smell of the ether during each surgery was sickening and sent me into hysterical fits. I remember the hospital staff, exerting great effort, pulling me screaming from my father's arms, and watching my mother and father peering through the round windows of the hospital doors as I disappeared down the hall to yet another surgery. I remember being racked with fear before my final surgery and nurses removing me from the children's ward to a room by myself. Restrained in the hospital bed, I spent the entire night sobbing uncontrollably, wishing the nurse that was standing guard by my bed would just come over for a moment and comfort me.

My seventh and final surgery to save my left eye occurred when I was four. Half-way through the surgery the doctor came to my parents with a medical consent form to sign. He had done all he could do and now he needed their permission to remove my eye. The surgeries for the left eye were now over. Everything medically that could be done had been exhausted. It was time for us to go home and adjust to life with my prosthetic eye.

When I was three, an unexpected addition came to the Valdez family: my younger brother, Robert, was born. Robert's arrival came to a family whose energies were focused on caring for a sick child. Mama Vicki and my mother's sisters did all they could to make up to Cathy and Robert for my mother's attention having to be focused on me. Surely at times my siblings must have felt some hurt and resentment. Cathy and Robert were young children who needed their parents' attention as much as any other children, but they were born into a family with a sick brother and would have to learn to adjust to the demands of that situation.

I had some vision in my remaining eye, but the doctors never actually determined how much. I spent my days like every other kid at that time, glued to the front of the television watching my favorite cartoon shows, "Captain Kangaroo," "The Mickey Mouse Club," and my all-time favorite, "Rocky and Bullwinkle." I was able to see with that one eye for the next few years, which I consider the greatest blessing of my life, because I remember everything I had the opportunity to see. I remember seeing blue skies and white puffy clouds, a sunrise, and the sun setting on the Pacific Ocean. I remember seeing colors, the stars in the sky, and a full moon at night. I remember the white blanket of snow in winter.

The most important thing I remember is that I saw myself. The last time I remember seeing myself was when I was six years old. It was my sister Cathy's First Holy Communion, and my brother and I were all decked out in sport coats and ties; mine was a blue coat and a red tie. Before we left the house, I snuck back to my mother's bedroom to get a really good look at myself in her full-length mirror. Obviously, I was very impressed with what I saw, because when my sister's godmother arrived and told me how handsome I was, I lifted my head, threw out my chest, and replied enthusiastically, "Yes, I am!"

My mom and dad never treated me differently than my brother and sister. When I needed discipline I received it. I had my share of household chores. Since I couldn't mow the lawn very well (my parents weren't too fond of the argyle pattern that resulted when I tried), my mother taught me how to keep a very clean and neat home. My chores were cleaning the bathrooms and vacuuming. My mother inspired me to become the first blind, Chicano Felix Unger of the barrio.

I loved playing outside like any of the other neighborhood kids, and my mom was like every other mom; she'd tell me, "Alex, you can go out and play, but be home before dark." I'd come in around noon and ask "Mom, is it dark yet?" I would get together after school with all my friends and play games like dodge ball (they really called it "Bomb the Blind Guy") and Hide and Seek. (I'd be it. The game would last a couple of days.) It was while playing football with neighborhood pals at the age of six that I received two direct blows with the football to my remaining eye. Afraid to tell my parents what had happened, I kept it secret until many years later. Since I hid the fact that I had been hit in the eye while playing, it wasn't until months later, when the vision in my good eye began to deteriorate, that the doctors examined me and found that I had a detached retina. The light-sensitive membrane at the back of my eye that processed the images focused on it by the cornea and lens had separated from its supporting layers. Although treatment is available to reconnect a detached retina, preventing the complete loss of vision, the condition must be diagnosed and treated immediately for the procedure to be successful. Because I had never mentioned the injury, quite a bit of time had passed before the problem was discovered.

After the diagnosis, the doctors weighed every available option they had to preserve the last bit of vision in my remaining eye. When they had examined all possibilities they brought my parents and me into the office to explain the choices. Surgeries for detached retinas were very long procedures at that time, and the chances of success were at best 50/50. Because of the length of the operation there was a very real chance that I would not survive the procedure. Without the operation I would eventually become totally blind. It was now up to my parents to make their decision. There I sat in the room with these three adults, listening to them discuss my fate, knowing what they were saying and yet not quite understanding what the future would hold for me.

My mother and father made a very difficult decision that day, but in my mind, their decision was the right one. My parents chose to take me home without anymore surgeries. We went home that day to begin my life as a child who was destined to become blind. No explanations were ever made to me, no child psychologists helped me deal with what was going to happen, and my parents and siblings did not participate in any support groups. We were off on this adventure alone.

My brother, Robert, would play an important role in my journey to reach a "normal" and independent life. Just three years younger than I, healthy and active, Robert would be the yardstick on which I would measure myself as I grew. He became my compadre, my nemesis, my protector, my antagonist. Anything Robert did or had, I had to do or have as well. When Robert played baseball, I played baseball; when Robert skate-boarded, I skateboarded; when Robert got a stingray bike and learned to ride, I did too. With a little reserva-tion my father succumbed to my unrelenting pleas and bought me my first bike. At this time we lived in a home that had a long, straight alley behind it. Down the center of this alley was a gutter, an indentation. I learned that if I stayed in the center of the gutter I could ride my bike by myself. From our house on the corner I could ride in a burst of speed the full length of the block then stop turn around and race back. It was great! If I felt myself going up the sides of the gutter I corrected my direction and came back to the center. That is the way I learned to ride a bike alone, just like Robert and his friends.

In school I was held back to repeat the first grade in order to adjust to my becoming blind. I remember learning to read Braille, all of those little white dots. I got so excited I ran home and read a stucco wall! While my parents' attitude was instrumental in giving me the confidence and drive to do anything I wanted, I still needed the skills necessary to live an independent life as a person without vision in a sighted world.

I was truly blessed by having a young, innovative, enthusiastic visual impairment teacher by the name of Annabel Schoof. Fresh from school and loaded with ideas, Miss Schoof laid down the academic cornerstones for me to lead a successful life. With a strong emphasis on the basics, including Braille reading and writing and tactile and audio skills, she taught her students the tools that would allow us to be mainstreamed and com-petitive in the public school system. She also had the foresight to teach us not only the tools we would need to get through our school years, but also skills that would allow us to live normal, independent lives as adults. Miss Schoof realized that as adults her students would be asked to sign their own names and she did not want them to have to sign an "x." In the third grade, when other students were learning cursive handwriting, Miss Schoof, with great patience, worked the entire year to teach each one of her students how to write his or her own signature. It is with great pride that when asked to sign a contract or check I can take out a pen and sign my name like everybody else. She also taught each of us how to use a manual typewriter so that we could communicate effectively on paper in a sighted world, a skill that has allowed me an easy transition to today's computer keyboard.

By the age of seven I was totally blind, unable to perceive light. To name the day that I became completely blind would be impossible, because the progression of my blindness over that year was so gradual that I did not even notice. It was not until I began bumping into things that I realized I had truly become blind. As the vision in my eye disappeared, my mind's eye took over. All the memory of the sights from the years that I could see replaced the vision my physical eye was losing. To explain this is difficult, but the images that I see have the appearance of coming from my right eye just the same as when I was able to see. While I do not understand how this is possible, I believe that the reason might be that I was born with a photographic memory. Although I am totally blind, I am a very visual person, and my life is full of color, images, and light, not darkness. I dream in images and color, my mind provides my sight as I go through each day. I consider myself very lucky to have had vision long enough to understand the concept of the third dimension of depth. This knowledge has been instrumental in the high level of mobility that I have been able to achieve. Because the visions I carry are from the 1950s, I have no concept of smog. My colors come from a 1950s crayon box so I do not understand fluorescents, and to me, most of the women I meet look a lot like Donna Reed or Wilma Flintstone.

After two years of living without vision a change began to occur in me. For a year when I was nine I became an extremely angry child and acted that anger out. While I have no memory of what brought on the change or exactly why I was angry, I do know I did not want to be blind. I asked my mother one day why this had happened to me, why not the neighbor kid that I didn't like, why me? Her response to my question was the only explanation she had to give, the answer was that it was God's will. From that moment I hated God. Why would He do this to me? Why not one of the other kids I knew? What had I done to deserve this punishment? It would be years and years before I could forgive God for what I believed He had done to me.

As my eye slowly deteriorated it took on a film of white discoloration that made me the object of teasing and taunting by other children. My brother, taking the role of my protector, would defend me, staring back at anyone, including adults, who had the nerve to stare, using his small body to block their view of me. My father taught me a different approach to deflect their cruel remarks. His solution was that when asked why my eye looked the way it did, I should tell them "It's because I have X-ray vision and right now I can see you have a hole in your underwear." It worked!

My father was the joker of the family and he passed on this wonderful gift of humor to me. It was not until I was in the third grade that I recognized the real power in humor. We were going to see a film in class. The teacher closed the drapes and turned off the lights. From my seat in the back row I yelled out, "Duck down, Marty, I can't see!" The classroom broke up and I was hooked. I had found a very powerful tool, laughter, to help me through the rest of my life. I have always found that when you are able to laugh at the difficulties that present themselves in your life, you are able to take the power out of them and they become much easier to overcome.

At the age of eleven my family discovered Services for the Blind, a newly formed organization whose purpose was to address daily living and social skills for school-age children who were blind or visually impaired. Prior to this time I was not acquainted with any blind adults. It was during my first summer with Services that I would meet and get to know my very first role model who was blind. His name was Gary Spangler and he worked at Services as the youth coordinator. He lived by himself in an apartment, had a girlfriend, and was like anybody else, just a really cool guy! I don't know that I ever sat down and thought I wanted to be like him, but knowing Gary taught me, on a subconscious level, that a person who was blind could live on his own and have a fully independent life. Gary did not teach me this lesson in words that I might have soon forgotten. He taught me in the example set by the life he lived, which had a lasting impression on me.

The summers with Services for the Blind were some of the best of my childhood. We had weekend camping trips, beach outings and, my favorite, wood shop. To this day I can still build a mean box! The best summer I remember was when a local company donated a few dozen walkie talkies to our organization. That summer, with the help of Girl Scout volunteers, we headed off to Santiago Park. Santiago is not a sissy neighborhood playground, it is a real, densely wooded park with a large riverbed running down the center, steep hills, and over twenty-three acres of land. Each of us received a code name. Our mission was to explore the park alone, armed only with a walkie talkie and a white cane. Our instructions were to check in to Gary at home base every fifteen minutes. As we were exploring we were to keep track of the sounds, smells, and noises of the terrain we were covering so that if we got lost they could send out one of the Girl Scouts from home base to find us. That day taught me how to determine which way was north, to pay attention to my surroundings and be able to describe them in detail, to protect and take care of myself, but most of all it taught me independence.

Learning proper social skills and behavior is an important lesson for everyone who wants to be successful in life, and I believe it is even more important for those of us who might have a disability that can tend to isolate us from others. We are already under people's scrutiny, and by not acquiring acceptable social skills we run the risk of even further isolation. When I was twelve my father, brother, and I were invited by my father's boss to go dove hunting on his ranch. Other fathers and sons from my father's company were also invited. The group ended up totaling fifteen people. After a morning of hunting we all settled down for lunch at Mr. Klug's ranch house for a sandwich, chips, and a bottle of soda. That evening when I was passing my parents' room, I overheard my mom and dad talking. My father was telling my mother how very proud I had made him that day at lunch. The entire group had been seated at one long table and I sat directly across from my father and brother. Unknown to me as the meal was served, every head at the table turned my direction and every eye focused on me. Every person at that table was waiting for me to reenact the opening scene from the *Miracle Worker*, where Helen Keller grabs handfuls of food off everyone's plates, shoving it wildly into her mouth like a mad animal. Instead, I politely picked up my sandwich and proceeded with lunch in a fashion that would make Emily Post and my father proud, never once dropping a crumb or spilling an ounce of my soda.

When I was in the eighth grade I had my first encounter with show biz. While I was growing up very few television shows included the role of a person with a disability, and those that did had the character portrayed by an able-bodied actor. However, a visionary couple by the name of Jack and Bonita Rather, the owners of Lassie Productions, had the foresight to produce an episode of "Lassie" that not only had a storyline about blind children, but cast blind children in the roles. After a week of preparation from my junior high drama coach, I landed the role of Steve. Four long days of shooting quickly indoctrinated me into the world of television.

The most enduring lesson I learned from my "Lassie" experience is that it might look, smell, and taste like a ham and cheese sandwich, but it doesn't matter how hungry you are, you never, never eat your prop. This lesson was taught to me by a frustrated prop man who had to stop filming while he scurried down the mountainside to replace the two ham and cheese "props" I had devoured. Before my debut in "Lassie" I had dreamed of becoming a lawyer, but once I had smelled the grease paint there was no turning back.

High school was great; I liked high school. It was in high school that I met a teacher who would have the greatest impact on how I valued my world and others, but most importantly how I valued myself. Mr. Zimmerman was my visual impairment teacher. He was also my friend and confidant. He was an educated, successful, independent, blind man. He had studied at Julliard and was a consummate violinist. It was my good fortune that he chose teaching as a profession. He taught me to value my abilities. For instance, when running for an office in student government, I was required to give a speech in front of the entire student body. In the question-and-answer session that followed, a student yelled out, "Yeah, well, how are you going to do that, you're blind?" The remark took the wind out of me. Mr. Zimmerman was in the audience that day and he approached me as I left the auditorium. "Alex," he told me, "the next time someone hits you with a question like that, you tell them, 'We are not here to judge people on their disability, we are here to judge them on their ability.' " I have never forgotten what he said that day.

While growing up I was very fortunate to have never been a target of prejudice because of my Hispanic heritage, but in high school I came head on with my first experience of prejudice because of my disability. I met and began going out with a girl from a church choir to which we both belonged. After a few dates her parents took her aside and told her that she could no longer see me because I was blind. They told her that if by chance we became serious about each other and one day married, I would be unable to support her and she would have to spend the rest of her life taking care of me. To avoid any future heartache she was forbidden to see me and we broke up. Their decision was one that hurt me very deeply at the time. Today when I think about what happened it makes me smile. I like to envision her parents sitting down on their couch, turning on their television, and there I am smiling back at them from the TV screen. They turn to each other and in unison exclaim, "Damn!"

I always enjoyed athletics and in high school I wrestled, studied martial arts, and I even remember one winter going snow skiing with my brother and some friends. We headed to the local mountains to do some night skiing. I figured skiing in the dark, I had the advantage.

When we got to the slopes, my brother suggested that we take the rope tow up the mountain and ski back down. He showed me how to take my poles, pick up the rope, tuck it under my arm, keep my ski tips up and ride the rope up the mountainside. I got in line, picked up the rope, tucked it under my arm, and took off like a bat out of hell, skiing over the three or four people who were standing in line in front of me. Everybody fell down; there were skis and poles everywhere. Some guy yelled out "What are you, blind?" and I replied, "Yeah!" After we got ourselves straightened out and untangled, my brother said, "Alex, don't give up, try it again, and don't worry, I'll be right behind you!" Once again I got in line, picked up the rope, tucked it under my arm, and took off up the mountain.

There I was in that cool, crisp, pine-scented air; I was doing it! I was going up the mountain, with the tips of my skis riding on the ends of the skis of the woman who had gotten on right in front of me. I yelled over my shoulder, "Robert, how's this?" . . . "Robert, how's this?" . . . "Robert!" And lo and behold I realized that I was all alone on the mountain with this woman. Now this part didn't bother me, but I had no idea where or when to get off. I had visions of me, the rope, skis, poles, everything just going into some big machine and being spit out on the other side of the mountain.

After the woman asked me to drop back off the ends of her skis, I said to her, "Excuse me, can you tell me when do we get off?" She said, "Sure, at the end." So I told her, "I'm blind." She said, "You're *what?*" I said, "I'm blind, when do I get off?" "*Now!*" she screamed. I hurled myself into the snow, and lay there face down, with skis and poles pointing in every different direction. From the bottom of the mountain I heard gales of laughter—it was my brother and our friends. They were laughing so hard that when they got to me, they fell down too. They said, "Alex, it was the greatest thing we have ever seen, you flopped in five different directions at one time. People in the lodge were making bets if you were going to survive or not." At the end of the night when I put my equipment away, everybody knew that the guy in the red windpants was blind and crazy.

During high school I became very involved in the music department. When I graduated, I enrolled in college as a music major. However, at the end of my third year of college I came to the realization I would never be more than an average musician. I left school with no idea of what I was going to do with the rest of my life. A friend came to me and said, "You know, Alex, you ought to try stand-up comedy. Just think about how many blind musicians are out there, but how many blind comedians are there? You can be the very first and only one!" His idea intrigued me, but I was still a little reluctant. After four weeks of his badgering and a promise that he would help me write my set, he convinced me to give it a try. For the next month we worked on developing five minutes of material. I went to the Comedy Store, a comedy club in Westwood, California, three times before I finally got the nerve to go up on stage.

On June 6, 1977, with butterflies the size of vultures

in my stomach, I walked on to the stage for the very first time. I sat down on a bar stool and said, "There is no use hiding it, you've probably noticed by now, I'm totally deaf." That one line drew a loud round of applause. But after the opening, I walked on every laugh they gave me. Instead of waiting to begin my next joke, I just rushed right in. My timing was poor because of my lack of experience and my nerves. My knees were shaking so hard that I almost fell over. Upon leaving the stage that first night, I said "This is it!" I walked away that night to a standing ovation and I knew I'd found my calling—until I went back the following evening and bombed.

After bombing I made the decision not to give up, to take that failure and use it as an education. Though I had used humor all my life to break down the walls of people's fears and misconceptions about blindness, I found the owner of the club where I had been performing at the open mike* nights for the last five months did not agree. One night as the owner sat in her office she turned on the closed circuit camera to the stage. It just so happened that I was performing when she flipped the switch. She walked down to the show room and told the comedian running the show, "We can't have this, this is not right, you have to tell him he cannot come back!" The club owner did not approve of a blind comedian on stage, particularly one who was making fun of his disability. As a result, I was banned from participating in their open mike night, or, shall I say, supposedly banned. The comedian who ran the open mikes was a guy by the name

---

*On an open microphone (mike) night, a club will open the stage to anyone who would like to perform. These events provide a chance to those people trying to get into comedy to try out their material on a live audience.

of Danny Mora. Danny and I had quickly become friends and over the five months I had been coming to open mikes, he had been offering tips and coaching me. Together we devised a little scheme: I hung around the club and when the owner left for dinner, Danny snuck me up to get my stage time.

This little scenario went on for about a year until Danny decided we were ready to come clean. He told the owner that he had a new comic that he wanted to showcase for her. He did not let her know who she was going to be seeing. As I performed, she turned to Danny and remarked, "He doesn't even look blind." She liked what I did that night and I became a club regular. With Danny's help and my perseverance, we were able to get the stage time necessary to develop my comedic skills, so that the owner was able to see me for my ability as a comedian, not for my disability of blindness.

I have found that if you find a positive perspective on being unique, that uniqueness can have tremendous advantages. I was able to take my blindness, something that originally some club owners felt would depress the audiences, and by treating it as something unique, giving it a different perspective, I was able to challenge the audience's idea of what a man who was blind could do. In doing so I was able to make my being blind not only entertaining, but at the same time enlightening.

While I received enthusiastic acceptance and support by the vast majority of my peers, there were occasions when the stage time I received was openly resented by other comedians. One comedian in particular felt that I was getting preferential time slots because I was blind and remarked angrily to me, "I'd be getting stage time too if I poked my eyes out." Of course I told him to "go right ahead!"

After about a year and a half in the business I was approached by a friend named Geri Jewell, who had cerebral palsy. Geri and I had met in an acting class at Fullerton College (in Fullerton, California, a suburb of Los Angeles) and became very good friends. She knew that I had been doing stand-up comedy for a while and thought that she too, might want to give it a try. I told Geri to get her material together and when she was ready I'd take her with me to the Comedy Store to give stand-up a try. Geri did great her first night and was welcomed with open arms. Thus, there were two stand-up comedians with disabilities out there and attitudes were beginning to change.

As with all careers, comedy has had its ups and downs. One particular down happened at a club in Cincinnati about fifteen years ago. While I was tossing sunglasses to the crowd in preparation for a bit called "Get blind with Alex!" I ventured just one step too close to the edge of the stage, landing belly down in the center of a front row table, with candles and drinks flying. Then with a recovery that remains a mystery to everyone present, including myself, I bounced backwards and landed flat on my feet back on stage. That had to be a first date the couple sitting at that table wasn't going to soon forget.

Despite a cold or even hostile reception at times, I have found most people in the entertainment industry are willing to take a chance where people from other professions might not be. My mentors include such entertainment giants as Steve Allen, who was kind enough to critique and suggest material for me; Pat Morita, who spent a great deal of effort helping me learn the physical movements and expressions necessary to perform my material; and Bill Dana, Uncle Bill, who has developed ideas for a sitcom he and I could work on together. The owners of the Comedy and Magic Club and the Laff Stop allowed me regular workout time at their clubs. Paramount Studios provided empty sets on their lot as training ground for Performing Arts Theater of the Handicapped (PATH), a troupe of aspiring disabled entertainers of which Geri Jewell and I were members. Talented actors and directors such as Ron Howard, Henry Winkler, and Tom Bosley donated their time and energies to encourage and direct PATH productions. For all those people who saw the ability in me and provided the encouragement and education for me to realize my dream, I will be eternally grateful.

At the time he was directing PATH productions, Tom Bosley was well known as Mr. Cunningham, costar of the weekly sitcom "Happy Days." Tom was asked to appear as a guest host on the popular comedy television show, "Evening at the Improv." He agreed with one stipulation—that he be allowed to bring a young, blind comedian he knew to be one of the talent for that week's show. The producer agreed, and with Tom's help I had my first appearance on "Evening at the Improv" and my very first shot at national television exposure.

After four years as a comedian, I got a big break and was given the job of house master of ceremonies (MC) at the Laff Stop in Newport Beach, California. I had a real job! It was during this time that I had the opportunity to meet and work with a lot of the comedians who are motion picture and television stars today. Gary Shandling, Jay Leno, and Robin Williams are just a few who willingly shared their time, support, and expertise in helping me to develop my comedy skills. But the most important thing to me was that these guys accepted me as one of their peers.

One night I was working as MC, I met a comedian by the name of Jim O'Brien. He and his partner were working the Laff Stop and I was really amazed by the impressions and sound effects Jim did. Jim and I quickly became friends and he suggested that I come along with them on the road. Packing up and leaving friends, family, and a life that I was comfortable with was not an easy decision for me to make, but in life we must challenge ourselves, move out of the comfort zone, and try new things. In 1981, I set out across country with Jim and his partner to pursue my goal of becoming a nationally known comedian.

When Jim and his partner split up, Jim and I decided that we would combine our talents and become the comedy team of O'Brien and Valdez, the most unique comedy team ever. In all the years of comedy there has been every combination of team imaginable, but Jim and I were, and continue to be, the first and only able/disabled team in the history of comedy: a sighted Irish guy from Chicago and a blind Mexican from California.

The demands of being a member of a comedy team are much greater than those I encountered as a solo act. Timing is of the utmost importance for a team. Learning the exact time and direction of visual responses without the benefit of sight was painstakingly slow. I have a deep sense of pride in that I often encounter people who have seen my partner and me perform on television and are honestly shocked to learn that I am blind. That they think I have vision is not because we have made any effort to disguise the fact that I am blind. From the very start we chose to be up front about it. My white cane is always with me, even on stage. What it does mean is that I am destroying their idea of what a blind person should look like and how he should behave.

As a result of the willingness and open-mindedness of the people I have mentioned and the change I was able to make in the public's perception of a comedian with a disability, doors of acceptance have been opened in stand-up comedy for others with disabilities. When I stepped on the stage at the Comedy Store in 1977, I became the first comedian in this country with a disability. In doing so I turned the knob and cracked the door for other comedians with disabilities to follow. Each barrier of resistance I met and overcame opened that door a little wider. Each audience that saw a funny comedian instead of a blind guy telling jokes pushed the door open even more. When Geri Jewell followed me in performing comedy she took the door and gave it another push. Each time audiences saw a wonderfully funny comedienne instead of a person with cerebral palsy telling jokes, Geri was able to open the door a little wider.

Over the years as each comedian with a disability has come to the stage, showcasing his or her own special talents, the passageway to the profession of stand-up comedy has been opened wider. In recent years Geri and I have been followed by some extremely talented comedians who happen to have disabilities. We had the honor of appearing with many of these comedians on the PBS special, "Look Who's Laughing," an award-winning documentary that featured the stage performances and private observations of six comedians with disabilities. To receive this kind of recognition for being a stand-up comedian with a disability is something that I would never have dreamed possible twenty years ago.

During the late 1980s comedy had its peak, and since that time there has been a constant decline in the number of comedy clubs. Along with the reduction of clubs and the number of jobs available, there has also been a flood of people wanting to do stand-up comedy. Because of supply and demand, not only are there fewer clubs and more competition, but salaries and reimbursed expenses for these jobs are at an all time low. When I am approached by people wanting to get into stand-up comedy, I always suggest that they look long and hard at the realities of the profession. Comedy might look fun and glamorous from the audience's perspective, but from the stage it is a real job in which you spend the majority of each year on the road living out of a suitcase. Very few comedians are able to make a living at it. The demands take you away from family and friends. But, if you have it in your blood, are willing to pay the price it requires, and most importantly have an alternative plan in your back pocket, my advice is to get out there and give it a shot!

In the eleven years Jim and I have been a team, we have traveled the country performing at comedy clubs and universities and appearing on countless radio and television shows. I have always enjoyed doing comedy and feel very blessed that I have been able to make a living at something that I love so much, but comedy as a business started to slow down and I reached a point in my life where I was becoming a little road weary. I wanted to reacquaint myself with friends and family. I wanted to sleep in my own bed. I wanted to spend the holidays at home. Along with these things, I also wanted to challenge myself again. I was sitting alone in a hotel room in St. Louis, Missouri, tired of the long tour I was in the middle of and wondering what direction I should take in my career, when the phone rang. I picked it up and heard the voice of Geri Jewell. Geri said, "Alex, I have been doing professional speaking for a few years, traveling the country telling my story. You have a story that needs to be told and you should be out there telling that story."

In September 1994, with Geri's help and encouragement, I embarked on a second career in the arena of professional speaking. To tell you that it was easy would be untrue. There were moments prior to my first speech that I was all but paralyzed by fear. Comedy was comfortable, it was all I knew. I was forty years old. Why did I think I needed to change directions now? The first time I walked to the podium to give a speech was in Tampa, Florida, to an audience of over 500 people. All of a sudden, there they were again, those vultures in my stomach. I managed to make it through my speech that day and, thankfully, all of the speaking engagements that have followed. By pushing forward I have been able to move past my fear, because it is only by putting your fears out front where you can see them clearly that you can face them and find they are just shadows of your imagination.

I have grown to love public speaking as much as comedy. It has been a pleasure and a privilege to share my ideas and stories with others. I have had the opportunity to speak to colleges, organizations, and corporations across this country. My greatest honor is that I was chosen to speak at the Justice Department's first Employee Disability Awareness Day. It meant a lot to me to meet the chief of the Equal Employment Opportunity Commission, Mr. James Perez, a long-time advocate of civil rights in this country. Believe it or not, there I was, a Mexican from southern California in the office of Louis Freeh, the director of the FBI, and I wasn't even being questioned.

While comedy and professional speaking have both provided me with many personal rewards, speaking has also given me a great deal of personal satisfaction. My first opportunity to see that what I was doing really mattered was at my fourth engagement. I was speaking to a large group in Reading, Pennsylvania. Unknown to me, about 50 percent of the audience were high school students with various disabilities. After my presentation I had the opportunity to spend some time talking with the students. I was approached by a young girl who told me that she was a senior in high school and that she was dyslexic. The past few years had been very difficult for her and she had made up her mind that she was going to drop out of high school. Then she heard me speak. She realized that it was going to be difficult, but she decided to stay in school, finish her senior year and graduate. I was overwhelmed. The fact that I had reached that one girl meant more to me than any standing ovation I had received in my life. I may have helped her summon up the courage to stay in school, but she helped me to gather the determination it would take to ride out the difficult times in a new profession.

Traveling thirty to forty weeks a year performing comedy for over sixteen years left me just about enough time to do a load of laundry and repack when I got home. While I will never regret the career choice I made, it has left me limited time to become involved with volunteerism and my community. Because I am able to make more of a living in professional speaking, I am now able to spend less time away from home. Slowing down has not only allowed me to spend more time with those I care about, but it is starting to offer me more time to devote myself to the causes that I believe in.

Last year (1996) I had the honor of being asked to join the Board of Directors of Blind Children's Learning Center, a local school that educates children who are blind or visually impaired and their families. The curriculum is designed to include an early intervention program for children aged six months to six years. I am the first board member to be appointed who is blind. I believe this association will allow me the opportunity to share with these children all of the wonderful tools I learned when I was young and provide a message of hope and reassurance for their parents. Because children usually live up to our expectations of them, we should always expect the best. Children, blind or sighted, can do anything in this world that they want, but only if they believe they can.

While comedy and speaking are very different forms of communication with an audience, I use both to relay the same idea. My message to audiences is that even though some of us might look a little different on the outside, on the inside we are all very much the same. We all have hopes, fears, pain, goals, all the range of human desires and feelings. On stage performing comedy with my partner, Jim, the message is subtle. I demonstrate this "sameness" in sketches and bits, and usually in a very short period of time the audiences have forgotten that I am blind. In speaking, my message is very clear and up front. I explain that we are the same and support my belief through my life stories. While comedy and speaking are the ways I pay my bills and put food on the table, it is my hope that my message about the abilities of all people isn't restricted to the ways I earn a living. I hope the style in which I live my life might prove to be a better education than anything I can say or do in front of a spotlight. As Gary Spangler and Mr. Zimmerman taught me, the best examples are not the words that were said but the lives that were led.

Being blind has more than its share of frustrations.

Everyone's life does. My biggest frustration has and continues to be transportation. The fact that I cannot go out to a car sitting in my driveway, open the door, put the key in the ignition, and go anywhere I want to is frustrating. I have traveled this country for sixteen years by myself, but when it comes to traveling in my own neighborhood, it is difficult at best. I believe there will come a day in my community when public transportation is accessible for all people, including those of us who are totally blind. Today it is not. I still rely on family and friends to get me where I need to go. It is not easy always asking for a ride, but it is a necessity for me so that I can continue to work. Because it is so important, I have learned to swallow my pride and ask. The number one thing that I value in my life is my independence, and transportation is one of the few avenues where I am unable to achieve freedom. The day that rapid transit is able to meet the needs of blind consumers will be a very happy, liberating day in my life and in the lives of all people who are blind.

I believe transportation is one of, if not the most, difficult issue persons with disabilities encounter on the road to independence. Because of this I have a goal of becoming more involved in addressing the problems disabled travelers encounter. I am currently working on developing a program to present to all areas of the transportation industry from local public transit to commercial airlines about what they can do to facilitate accessibility of their particular form of transportation to the traveler with a disability.

I am also in the process of developing a program to teach school-age children about disability and diversity awareness. In reviewing curricula for school-age children I have noticed that there is very little attention given to educating children about the abilities of people with disabilities. Because young children are so very open and inquisitive it is to our benefit to open their minds and attitudes while they are young. A friend of mine took her five-year-old son grocery shopping with her. As she was selecting her purchases from the shelf she noticed her son staring at a gentleman in a motorized wheelchair. She put her things down and went to reprimand her son for staring. Before she could make her way to him, he ran to the side of the man in the chair. With a booming voice and the innocence of a child he inquired of the man, "Hey, mister, does that thing come with a remote?"

When I speak I tell my audiences about how I have used courage to rise above life's challenges and disappointments. I believe that in most people's minds the only time people are courageous is when they are on a battlefield with bullets whizzing above their head, or when they are being pulled down raging rapids while swimming furiously for shore, or perhaps even when blind people face lanes of swift traffic with only a white cane. I explain to them that every one of us can be courageous in our lives. Courage is very simple. Courage is nothing more than a positive mental attitude combined with action and supported by faith.

In my life my father taught me to use humor to keep a positive attitude no matter how difficult things became. My teachers, role models, and service organizations were the keys to learning the skills necessary to take action. My mother and Mama Vicki taught me the valuable lesson of keeping faith no matter how dark things might look at the moment. By using these three tools I have been able to meet the challenges in my life and use them as stepping stones to a better life. These are the same tools that anyone can use to reach his or her highest potential. The next time you see someone in a wheelchair or walking with a white cane, stop and remember, disabilities are sometimes more than meet the eye. While some people's disabilities may make them look very different on the outside, on the inside we are all very much the same!

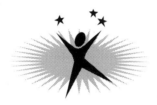

The Beauty Within

Michael Crisler

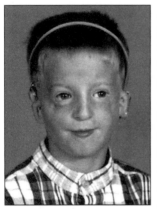

Michael Crisler, age seven, suffers from Treacher Collins Syndrome, a birth defect that causes the bones in the face to develop improperly. He has raised over $57,000 for different causes and charities, including more than $40,000 for the Oklahoma City bombing victims. He has also helped raise funds for many local and national charities, including Children's Miracle Network and the Muscular Dystrophy Association. He has received many awards but believes "it is better to give than receive." Michael also enjoys showing others that kids can make a difference in the world.

I have a birth defect called "Treacher Collins Syndrome." My cells didn't come together right when my body was forming, which prevented the bones in my face from developing as they should. Treacher Collins is a genetic condition, which means that one or more genes are either not working correctly or are not working at all. It can be as mild as a small bone missing where no one would notice, or so severe that a person's jaw is set back too far, requiring a trachea tube to breathe. Cleft lips and palates are very common results of this birth defect, and the heart can also be affected.

I was born with a cleft palate and missing cheek

bones, so the doctors used parts of my ribs to fill out my cheeks. My ears are very tiny; they did not grow bigger with the rest of my body. I do not have any ear canals so I wear a bone conduction hearing aid to hear. I am eight years old and have had five surgeries to restructure my face and expect to have at least twelve more.

Treacher Collins is usually inherited, which means that one of my parents has the same problem with their genes. I inherited Treacher Collins Syndrome from my mother, who was the first in our family history to have the disease. Her doctor said that in her, Treacher Collins was caused by a "spontaneous mutation"—the genes just changed and didn't work properly for some unknown reason. Now that she has it, though, it is hereditary and I have a 50 percent chance of passing this syndrome to my children. Since Treacher Collins affects the face, the defects are usually visible and therefore people, especially other children, tend to treat you a little differently.

Because I was born with this defect I feel like it's a part of my life and that I was made this way for a special purpose. Since I was born this way, it is not usually difficult for me to handle. If a child or adult asks my mom what is wrong with me, or why my face looks different, my mom always tells them to ask me directly. I gladly show them my hearing aid and demonstrate how the sound turns into vibrations. I let them feel what I hear. I try to explain my birth defect to them. Mom and I usually try to talk to anyone who has questions, and we often talk at conferences to try and make a difference in how people look at birth defects.

Sometimes when people (especially kids) tease me it really hurts my feelings and I feel sad. I always remember that my mom taught me not to tease anyone because you could be all right now, but you never know about tomorrow. You could be in an accident or become sick. Even Superman (Christopher Reeve) isn't perfect. While riding a horse Christopher Reeve fell and broke his neck. Now he is paralyzed from the neck down and he has to have help doing everything, even breathing. If this can happen to Superman, it can happen to anyone.

Mom always says that the more people know, the more they understand and the less attention they pay to someone's disabilities (and the less likely they are to tease). I believe that if you can't look past the outside to the inside of a person, then you are the one with the disability. People are like books. Just because the cover of the book is worn, stained, or looks terrible doesn't mean the book is a bad one. The only difference is the cover. Just like books, our covers are different but we're all just the same on the inside. I also feel that if you can learn to laugh at yourself, you can accept yourself as you are and not try to be something you're not.

For as long as I can remember, my mom and grandparents have always taught me how helping others can bring special joy, like no other feeling in the world. I realize that not everyone is as lucky as I am. I remember feeling sad for a little girl who lost her teddy bear in the big flood in the Midwest when her house floated away. I went up to my room and saw all of my teddy bears and decided to pick one out to give to her. Then I started wondering about all the other children who lost their bears. I packed up some of my other bears and insisted that my mom drive me to the television station that was taking donations to help the victims so I could deliver the boxes myself and give the station the one special bear I had picked out for the little girl I saw on television.

Many times at Christmas my mom, grandparents, and I adopt a family for the holiday and provide everything, including food, for them. I wrap some of my own toys to give to the children so that they can have more toys to open at Christmas.

My mother started me bowling when I was two and a half years old and I have always enjoyed it. I now bowl on several different teams and in tournaments. After I started bowling I began a bowl-a-thon for the Children's Miracle Network (CMN), a national organization started by Marie Osmond that has grown to be the largest annual television fundraiser in the country. The money raised by CMN stays in the community where it was donated. For example, money raised in Colorado goes to the National Jewish Hospital in Denver. It felt so good trying to help sick children, especially since some of the money was used for research to help the children get better. I have been the top fundraiser in Colorado for the last three years and I plan to continue to be the top fundraiser in the state and maybe even the nation in the future! I also help raise money for the Muscular Dystrophy Association by participating in a bowl-a-thon (I have raised the most money in our bowling alley for the past two years). Nothing can match the feeling in my heart when I know that something I have done is helping other people.

I watched the children suffering after the Murrah Federal Building was bombed in Oklahoma City on April 19, 1995, and I felt like I had to do something. I felt so sad for the grown-ups who lost their kids and the kids who lost their moms and dads. I sympathized with all those children and adults who were hurt—I know what it feels like to be in the hospital and it is no fun. Since I had just finished a bowl-a-thon for the Children's Miracle Network, I asked my mom if she would let me do another bowl-a-thon to raise money for the victims of the bombing. When she first asked me how much I wanted to raise, I said $20,000. She asked me to be more realistic because she didn't think that I could raise that amount, so I changed my goal to $10,000. Mom tried to get me to lower it to $5,000, but I refused. Mom gave me her permission but said I would have to go to the bowling alley and ask the manager for his. That night, Mom and I made a flyer to show the manager my idea. The next morning I looked at the flyer and noticed something different. I realized that my mom had changed the goal to $5,000. I got very upset even though Mom said she did it because she was afraid that I might not be able to raise the $10,000 and she didn't want me to be disappointed. Determined, I changed the number back to $10,000 and told her that if we get enough good people to help we could make our goal and really help the people in Oklahoma City. Ten thousand dollars would help twice as many people as $5,000 would. I put on my three-piece suit and asked Mom to drive me to the bowling alley. I was very happy when the manager agreed to help us.

The people at the bowling alley helped me set up the bowl-a-thon and helped me contact the media. Channel 4 KCNC-TV, a CBS station, came out to interview me before the bowl-a-thon and said that they would bowl (they ended up donating $500). Then lots of other people started calling in to bowl. My mom drove me from door to door to different businesses to ask for sponsors. Because of everyone's cooperation the bowl-a-thon was very successful. We had forty or so people bowl and several television stations covered the event. A lot of people also just sent donations to our house. Before we knew it my mom said that we had raised over $27,000.

Governor Frank Keating of Oklahoma invited me

and my family to Oklahoma City to deliver the money. I wanted all of the money to go to the victims and their families, so Governor Keating set up a fund so that would happen.

We had originally planned to drive to Oklahoma with my grandparents in their motorhome. Then channel 4 and channel 9 (KUSA-TV, an NBC station) and *People* magazine wanted to go with us. Channel 4 arranged it with an airline to fly us to Oklahoma City so all of the media could go with us.

The meeting with Governor Keating was real neat, although it was really hard with all of the media attention—all the lights and the questions. I don't raise money for publicity. I feel that God wants me to do this and I have always believed it is better to give than receive. But I guess I should have been used to it; it was the same way when I was invited to Governor Roy Romer's office in Denver. Walking through the capital was really neat too. The media asked me which governor I liked the best. I said both.

When we got back to Denver I couldn't believe the money and cards that were still coming to our house. Mom and I sent another check to Governor Keating, bringing the total to $36,648. I hoped it would reach $40,000 by the end of 1995, but I don't think we reached quite that amount.

My life has been crazy since we came back from Oklahoma. My school had a "Michael Crisler Day" and everyone wore badges that said "I can make a difference just like Michael." We had a school program that included honoring all of the other kids and showing how they made a difference. The Oklahoma governor and Senate sent a proclamation and declared July 31 Michael Crisler Day. I received a proclamation from the

Englewood City Council (a suburb of Denver) and was formally recognized in the Colorado House of Representatives and the Senate.

I received a very nice letter and picture from President Bill Clinton. Shortly after I had reconstructive surgery on my face in the summer of 1996, I helped carry the torch to kick off the thirty-day countdown until the Olympic Festival with Governor Romer at the Colorado Rockies baseball game. They let me throw out the first pitch.

I also received an award from the Salvation Army, who invited me to be the Grand Marshall of their fifteenth annual Parade of Lights. I received the first annual Starlight Award, which honors youngsters who are making a difference by helping others and, in the spirit of giving, to inspire other children and families to make community service a part of their own lives. In addition the Salvation Army donated a $100 savings bond and they donated $100 to the Michael Crisler Fund for children in need (my church set up the fund so I can always help other children).

The most satisfying reward I ever got was when I was in the hospital recovering from surgery and my mother got a phone call from a woman who wanted to thank me. She said that she had an eleven-year-old son named Tyler who had Treacher Collins Syndrome. The neighborhood kids had tormented him since he was little and they wouldn't play with him. After I appeared on television the kids realized that if I was like a "normal" kid then Tyler must be okay and they started playing with him. This really made me feel good. It was better then all of the other awards put together.

I really wanted to prove to the world that even a child, no matter what is wrong with him, can make a difference. If everyone, adults *and* children, would do one thing to make a difference in this world, we could all make it a much better place to live.

I think my family is the most important part of my life. They have helped make me into what I am today. God is also very important to me. But most important to me is that people learn to live with each other, even with all their differences.

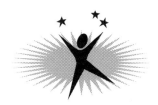

A Friend Can Make the Difference

Roxanne Black

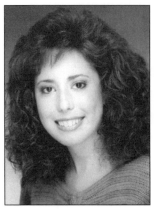

Roxanne Black was diagnosed with systemic lupus at the age of fifteen. She started Friends' Health Connection, a worldwide network that connects people who have the same health problems on a customized, one-to-one basis so they can communicate for the purpose of mutual support. More than 4,000 people across the country and around the world have joined Friends' Health Connection. Among other honors, she was named in Ladies' Home Journal's *Salute to American Women and most recently was honored by Governor Christie Todd Whitman of New Jersey.*

Eleven years ago, at the age of fifteen, I was diagnosed with lupus, a chronic autoimmune disease that can cause inflammation of various parts of the body, especially the skin, joints, and kidneys. For most people, lupus is a mild disease, but for others, it may cause serious and even life-threatening problems.

My diagnosis was a shock: I had always been healthy and suddenly my life was completely transformed as I began suffering severe joint pain, back pain, and inflammation. After I was released from the hospital, I was tutored at home because I was too weak to return to school. The main questions I continued to ask were

"Why me? What did I do to deserve this?" But there were no answers, reasons, or explanations.

The years that followed were filled with difficulties. I endured many of the typical lupus symptoms and experienced countless side effects from medications. Achy joints, arthritis, pleurisy,* fatigue, hair loss, and weight gain became a central part of my everyday life.

I wanted very much to talk to other people who also had lupus, so I decided to establish a support group in my area. However, since I was diagnosed with the disease at an uncommonly young age, I was the youngest member in the group and my needs were different than the older members'. For example, during meetings, we would discuss the impact of lupus on a marriage, but no one could relate to how I felt about enduring the pain and side effects of medications while attending high school. I started to look for another lupus teenager who could understand what I was experiencing, but my search was unsuccessful.

I knew that other people with health problems must have the same feelings of loneliness and isolation that I did, and that gave me an idea. During my freshman year of college I decided to form a network to connect people who are the same age and who have the same health problems on a one-to-one basis so they can communicate for the purpose of mutual support. Rather than limit this network only to lupus patients, I decided that anyone of any age with any type of health problem would be welcome to participate. I titled my program Friends' Health Connection (FHC) and I began working

---

*Pleurisy is a condition in which the membrane that lines the chest and covers the lungs becomes inflamed, causing pain on breathing.

out of my tiny dorm room at Rutgers, the State University of New Jersey.

At the time, my goal was to begin a small, statewide organization. However, as a result of considerable media coverage over the past six years, the group has grown nationally and internationally. To date, more than 4,000 people from across the country and around the world have joined Friends' Health Connection. Members include children, teenagers, adults, and senior citizens. Their health problems range from the most common to very rare disorders. We connect people whose overall situations are as similar as possible. Participants are networked according to their health problem, age, and other criteria such as symptoms, medications, surgeries, current stage of the health problem, attitude toward the health problem, occupation, hobbies, and interests.

All in all, Friends' Health Connection's network of people helping people strives to ensure that every person facing a health problem has a friend who understands and is willing to help guide the way and/or share the journey. Isolation is alleviated and renewed hope is often instilled in the hearts of members. The emphasis is placed on highlighting one's ability rather than dwelling on the inherent problems of coping with a serious illness or disability, thus helping participants to achieve and maintain a vital, positive attitude. This mutual inspiration often empowers both parties with the inner determination and positive attitude needed to continue fighting against illness.

During my sophomore year of college, lupus destroyed my kidney function, forcing me to administer dialysis to myself five times a day for nearly two years. Although I discussed the dialysis with friends and family members, I could not explain how it felt to go home between classes, connect myself to a bag for a half hour, and then leave in time for the next class; or end a date early because I knew if I didn't get home to administer the dialysis in time, I would feel ill. I could not fully express my fears about the future and the effects of dialysis on a job or a marriage and children. Worst of all, how could I accept my limitations—my lack of independence and my loss of freedom? I couldn't.

That is why Friends' Health Connection is so important. Regardless of the support a patient might receive from family members or friends, there is *no* way anyone who has not been there can understand what an individual feels. Until you lose your kidney functions, you cannot even imagine what it feels like to be connected to a dialysis machine. Until you are placed on a waiting list for an organ transplant, you cannot comprehend the tension that accompanies your every move.

Through Friends' Health Connection a patient can find people who can honestly say "I understand." A patient does not need to explain how he feels or what he fears because he is dealing with others who have experienced the same things, both physically and emotionally. Through Friends' Health Connection, a patient can find a friend—someone who can make the difference between acceptance and denial, the difference between fighting on and giving up, the difference between positive and negative. And sometimes the difference between life and death.

Friends' Health Connection has been featured in media both across the country and around the world. The organization has been praised by more than two dozen prominent individuals and organizations. In October 1990, President George Bush named me his 268th

Daily Point of Light,* and, in 1991 I was one of eighteen college students named to *USA Today*'s All USA College Academic Team. But more important than the awards are the many letters of gratitude that are continuously sent to FHC from members who have benefited from the program.

One story that comes to mind centers around thirty-one-year-old Maria, who was diagnosed with lupus. After her diagnosis, Maria thought that she could never have children. Friends' Health Connection paired Maria with Janet, another FHC member with lupus who had three healthy children. Janet convinced Maria that she *could* have children despite the disease. Since they began corresponding five years ago, Maria has given birth to two healthy, gorgeous sons. The women finally met face-to-face last year on ABC TV's "Mike & Maty" show.

Thirty-year-old Jennifer has chronic fatigue syndrome and endometriosis. For nine years, doctors have been telling her that a laparoscopy and cystoscopy† would help reduce her pain. Friends' Health Connection put Jennifer in touch with Samantha, who had already been through these surgeries. They talked on the telephone, discussing the risks and benefits of undergoing the procedures. Together they finally decided it should be

---

*The Daily Point of Light recognition was an honor bestowed by President Bush on those who performed outstanding acts of service. A different recipient was chosen each day that Bush was in office.

†*Endometriosis*: a condition in which endometrial tissue, the inner layer of the uterine wall, occurs outside the uterus, frequently resulting in the formation of cysts. *Laparoscopy* and *cystoscopy*: procedures in which the contents of the abdominal cavity and bladder, respectively, are examined by creating small incisions and inserting the correct type of endoscope, a lighted, tubular instrument that allows the doctor to view the interior of various organs.

done and Samantha helped Jennifer prepare herself emotionally. Since the surgeries, Jennifer feels much better and she now refers to Samantha as her sister. They met face-to-face several years ago on "Have a Heart," a television show produced by America's Talking.

Twenty-three-year-old Keith had a severe eating disorder. He joined FHC at a weight of seventy-five pounds. He was put in touch with Debbie, an FHC member who had overcome a severe eating disorder. Since corresponding with his FHC friend, Keith has virtually overcome his bulimia and his binges and purges rarely occur. He now weighs more than one hundred pounds.

These are just a few of the many members who have been helped by Friends' Health Connection. Whether they have made a major life change, gone ahead with a surgery, or learned through example, their stories help to confirm FHC's overall premise: *A friend can make the difference.*

Due to the growing number of requests from relatives of patients, Friends' Health Connection's Family Network was established two years ago to network relatives and friends of people with health problems. The family network connects siblings, spouses, parents, children, grandparents, and anyone else who is related to someone with a health problem.

Family Network has proven to be extremely beneficial to parents of babies born with birth defects and in cases where a spouse becomes the caretaker, as with Alzheimer's patients and with family members of individuals who have debilitating, chronic, and life-threatening disorders. One good example is Melissa, age twenty-five, whose mother has been battling cancer for several years. Melissa found strength, hope, and answers from Julie, her FHC friend, who was there to listen and support her throughout her most difficult days. Melissa met Julie face-to-face this year when they were brought together on Oprah Winfrey's television show.

After I graduated from Rutgers University in 1992 I received a grant from Johnson & Johnson so I could continue Friends' Health Connection. Since then, FHC has received additional funding from various other corporations and foundations and this has enabled us to establish a national telephone hotline that anyone with a health problem can call in order to become a member of Friends' Health Connection. We have also been able to unite Friends' Health Connection with major hospitals. The host hospitals publicize FHC to their patients through posters, information tents, flyers, buttons, stickers, and brochures distributed throughout their facilities. Gradually, we intend to implement the program in many other hospitals on a national level. By bringing the program to hospitals, FHC is able to reach patients at a time when emotional support is most critical.

During my senior year of college, my oldest sister, Bonnie, donated her kidney to me. After the transplant I felt stronger than ever. And, even though the doctors had previously thought I was headed for a wheelchair, the nerve damage caused by dialysis miraculously reversed itself. After the transplant I returned to college and was able to graduate the following month.

Today, I can finally answer the question I had asked myself so many times before: "Why me?" I now believe I became ill so I could help others. Today I can look back and realize that the lessons I have learned from my experiences are priceless. In addition to improving my intellectual capacity, they have influenced me socially and taught me where my priorities should lie. I have learned about the struggle that life entails and endured the

pressure and surprises that are a part of life. In addition, I now know that if there's a strong enough will
then there's a possible way. I've also discovered that although they are not always apparent, there are underlying reasons for everything. Underneath the pain, suffering, and despair lies a hidden opportunity to turn a
seemingly unfortunate circumstance into a situation
that is beneficial for oneself and for humankind.

You can join Friends' Health Connection by calling our
toll-free phone line at 1(800)48–FRIEND [1(800)483–
7436] or by visiting our web site at http://www.
48friend.com.

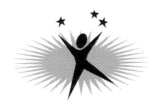

A Retreat from Asylum:
Finding My Place in the Real World

Paige Barton

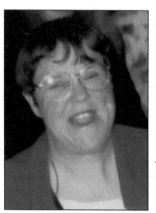

Paige Barton suffers from Trisomy 18, a genetic disorder which kills 90 percent of its victims between birth and age five. Due to the physical effects of the disease, she was misdiagnosed with Down's Syndrome and from the age of fifteen to thirty she was placed in institutions for the mentally retarded. After receiving her B.A., Paige began her mission to educate the public about the disabled and issues that affect them. She currently works for the Department of Mental Health, Mental Retardation, and Substance Abuse Services of the State of Maine, where she is Program Coordinator for people with developmental disabilities. Paige speaks nationally and founded a statewide conference for the disabled that draws hundreds of people annually.

I was diagnosed with Down's Syndrome at birth. At that time, there were no tests available to identify Down's, so the doctors based their diagnosis on the way that I looked. My parents were told that I was a mongoloid.

Down's Syndrome is a genetic condition that affects the twenty-first chromosome. Normally, people have twenty-three pairs of chromosomes, two in each pair. When someone has Down's, he or she has three chromosomes on the twenty-first pair instead of two. People with Down's Syndrome are very often mentally retarded, have heart defects, hearing loss, slanted eyes, and very small fingers.

For the first fifteen years of my life I lived at home and attended public schools. The kids at school always picked on me and called me names. I was slower at catching on to things than other students and some of the teachers weren't very patient with me. After seeking help and finding none, my mother didn't know what to do. She asked our family doctor and the principal at my school for advice. They told her to put me in an institution and leave me there for the rest of my life. My mother came to school one day and told me to clean out my locker because I wouldn't be coming back to school. I didn't know what was happening, or why, but I figured my mother knew what was best for me.

Three days later I was on my way to the first of six different institutions. I was sent to a crippled children's home, then a mental hospital, two group homes, a foster home, and finally a mental retardation center, all of which were located in Pennsylvania and Ohio. Twenty-five years ago, our society dealt with people who have Down's Syndrome and other afflictions by sending them to institutions. As Dr. Paul LaMarce, a retired geneticist, recently commented on the "Today" show, "institutions were just warehouses for the mentally retarded. There was no support to help families keep their children at home."

Although my family knew my diagnosis when I was seventeen months old, I did not learn what was wrong with me until I was thirty-two. I knew I was different but I didn't know how or why. I thought I was mentally retarded because I had been institutionalized with

people who were. When I was thirty-two, I found out, literally by accident, that I had been diagnosed as having
Down's Syndrome. At that time I was recovering from
having been hit by a truck and I went to see a lawyer
about how to get the bills from the accident paid for. The
lawyer told me that my brother had informed him that
I had Down's Syndrome, but that was the first time that
I had ever heard those words. I didn't know what they
meant. I went to the nursing home where I worked and
one of the nurses explained the meaning of Down's Syndrome to me.

My feelings at the time were mixed. I was glad that I
finally knew what was wrong with me, but I was also
angry that my family hadn't told me when I was younger.
If I had been told as a child, I would have been better
able to deal with the kids at school picking on me and
calling me names. It would have also helped me understand why I was placed in the institutions.

My feelings while I was in the institutions were ones
of fear, anger, confusion, and loneliness. I had been
taken away from my family and friends and I couldn't
understand why. The institutions "handled" me by
keeping me drugged with medication or giving me shock
treatments. I missed my family and friends and was
scared I would never get out of those places. In the beginning I didn't think I belonged there, but as time went
on I began to believe I did. Because I was living with
people who acted a certain way, I picked up some of their
behavior. For example, I saw people on the staff who
would only respond if you swore at them, so I started
swearing.

While I was in the institutions I began to work with
children who were severely retarded as part of the Patient Aid Program. We would feed the children break-

fast, clean them up, and then feed them lunch. I enjoyed helping out and in the last institution I was trained to work as a housekeeping aid in a nursing home.

In 1975 Public Law 94–142 was passed, stating that all people should receive an education in the least restrictive environment. In other words, each child deserves to receive an education in a public school (not an institution) designed to accommodate his ability to learn. This law also led to retesting the IQ of people who were institutionalized. When they retested me they said, "You have got to get out of here." A lady who was working with me at the nursing home took me in as a foster child and I lived with her for two years. In 1978 I took the test for my general education diploma and passed.

In 1980, when I was twenty-nine, I moved to Maine because my parents and brother had moved there while I was in the institutions. I wanted to be closer to my family but free from the institutions, group homes, and foster homes. I just wanted to live a normal life. I moved to Pittsfield and lived with my brother for one month. My parents thought I should move to Kennebunkport, where they were living, but I knew if I moved back home with them they would just place me in another institution.

After living with my brother I got a job working as a live-in housekeeper for a retired dentist, a post I held for three years. Then I moved to Farmington, where I worked as a housekeeping aide at a nursing home for two years.

In the fall of 1985 I entered the University of Maine at Farmington (UMF) to begin studying for my associate's degree in Early Childhood Education. I had taken a couple of classes and always dreamed of working with young children in a daycare center or nursery school. I knew that in order to do that I would need to further my

education. In the process of getting my degree many
things happened to me. I met some very special children
with disabilities. Their parents wanted to have the kids
mainstreamed into regular daycare and nursery
schools, but no school would take them because no one
had been trained to work with children with disabilities.
The university recognized this lack, and to remedy the
problem, a steering committee (which I joined) was created to develop an appropriate degree program.

In May 1987, I received my associate degree and
began working on my bachelor's in Early Childhood Special Education, even though the program wasn't fully
developed yet. In January 1989, UMF became the first
college in Maine to offer an undergraduate program in
Early Childhood Special Education.

In the fall of 1986 I attended a Bible and life retreat
with the Intervarsity Christian Fellowship. The lord really touched me at the retreat and said He had something He wanted me to do. I prayed "Lord, whatever you
want, you're going to have to show me what it is." I was
back from the retreat only one day when a lady came in
the snack bar where I was eating lunch. She introduced
herself as Joanne Petnam. Joanne was the chairperson
of the Special Education Department at UMF and knew
a lot about Down's Syndrome. She wanted me to talk to
others about my experiences with Down's. At first, I
didn't think that I could get up and speak in front of
people, but I knew I would find the strength I needed to
do this. I had been given a talent and I should use it.

I began by speaking to Joanne's classes at the university. I was very nervous at first, but each time I spoke
I became more confident. Joanne and I submitted a proposal to the National Down Syndrome Congress for me
to be a presenter at their national conference. They ac-

cepted our proposal and in November 1987, I spoke at my first national conference.

With Joanne's encouragement I decided it was time to have the diagnostic blood test for Down's Syndrome, which I had never taken before. The blood test came back normal and I didn't know what to think. I knew there was something wrong with me, but wasn't sure what it was. After many X-rays and a tissue test in January 1988, I found out that I actually have Trisomy 18 Mosaicisum.

When I first found out I had Trisomy 18 I was relieved. I finally knew exactly what was wrong with me. I was also angry because fifteen years of my life had been taken away by an incorrect diagnosis of Down's Syndrome. And I was also scared—in the beginning neither Joanne nor I could find any information about Trisomy 18.

After much research I discovered that Trisomy 18, like Down's, is a chromosome disorder. It affects the eighteenth chromosome whereas Down's affects the twenty-first. For people with Trisomy 18, I am writing medical history: I'm the oldest person alive with the disorder. Ninety-five percent of children born with Trisomy 18 die before they reach their fifth birthday. Most of those who live longer can't walk or talk. Trisomy 18 often affects eyesight, hearing, the heart, kidneys, and lungs. Many people require feeding tubes and children with Trisomy 18 are often mentally retarded. Only 7 percent of my cells are affected by Trisomy 18 (the word "mosaicisum" in the name of my disease means only part of my cells are affected), and this is why I have been able to live as long as I have.

In June 1988, another very encouraging thing happened in my life. I learned about Support Organization for Trisomy 18 (SOFT), a support group for people with Trisomy 18 and other related disorders. I went to my first SOFT Conference in July 1988 and I returned from the conference with a better understanding about Trisomy 18 and all of the things that are wrong with me. I learned at the conference that my 50 percent hearing loss, my recurrent respiratory problems, and my weak kidneys are the result of the disease. I also left the conference with a wonderful support network to help me through some of the things that happen, like problems that have arisen with my legs and possible Trisomy 18-related diabetes. I am also able to help families who have lost their children to this disorder just by remembering their birthdays and the date they died. I send the families a card or call them and just let them know I am thinking about them. This is one small way I can give back some of the support the group gives me.

My feelings toward learning I had Trisomy 18 have evolved from my initial reactions of anger and anxiety. Now I see myself as a walking, talking miracle. To me, Trisomy 18 is a death sentence. I am the oldest person alive who has it and I don't know how long I will live. Whenever I have new medical problems my doctors must try to figure out whether they are related to Trisomy 18.

I think the most difficult thing for me is all the things that are happening with my legs. Until four years ago, I could run, jump, and walk just like anyone else, but I now have to use a cane or wheelchair to get around. I can't climb stairs, which sometimes makes it very difficult. The nerves in my knees and legs aren't very strong and sometimes my legs give out on me. I have to wear high-top shoes all the time and I fall when I try to walk without assistance. I have undergone physical therapy and the exercises have helped me, but it's still a struggle.

The doctors believe that this degeneration in my legs is related to Trisomy 18, but because there is no basis of comparison (no one else with Trisomy 18 has lived as long as I have), they can't be sure. I'm in constant pain and have very bad muscle spasms. The doctors have tried various types of pain medication but nothing has worked. I can only hope that someday we will find something that will work. Until then I just keep a positive attitude and keep doing the best that I can.

I was encouraged to help others who have had the same or similar experiences as mine by some very special friends and by my faith. I can help people with disabilities see beyond their labels and help them speak up for themselves. We need to educate parents, doctors, teachers, professionals, and people in government to stop putting limitations on us because of our disabilities and to see us as people first.

After graduation from UMF in May 1991, I began looking for a job. I had a Bachelor's degree in general studies* and wasn't sure where to look for work. In the summer of 1990, I completed an internship with the Maine State Department of Mental Retardation. Through that program I traveled throughout the state. I had done some self-advocacy work helping people learn to speak up for themselves and visited several programs

---

*Although my plan had been to get my degree in Early Childhood Special Education, my grade point average was not high enough for me to student teach, so I switched programs and completed my degree in general studies. This actually turned out to be a blessing because my deteriorating knees and legs would have precluded me from the jobs in daycare and nursery schools for which the Early Childhood degree would have qualified me.

that provided services to adults with mental retardation and developmental disabilities. A man I had met at a conference in 1990, Dick Tryon, the executive director of Community Support Services, Inc. (CSSI), told me he might be able to help me find a job. Community Support Services, Inc., my employer, is a nonprofit agency that provides a wide range of services including residential facilities and vocational and day programming* to adults with mental retardation and developmental disabilities. They have a variety of homes including intermediate care facilities, nursing homes, Medicaid waiver homes, supported living apartments, and independent living. They also have a day program that provides services such as vocational training; speech, physical, and occupational therapy; and daily living skills instruction. CSSI has several job sites in the community and runs a retail store. Altogether they provide services to two hundred people.

In August 1991, I started working as a consultant for CSSI, organizing support groups for people who wanted to move out of group homes and into their own apartments. When I first started, I was only able to get three to five hours of work a week, but in January 1992, CSSI was able to acquire funding to expand my job to twenty hours a week. This allowed me to work more with the legislators on funding issues that affected people with developmental disabilities. In May 1992, CSSI created a job for me as a self-advocacy organizer. At first I worked twenty hours a week at CSSI and twenty hours a week as a worksite aide at one of the job sites, but the self-advocacy organizer position became a

---

*Day programming involves part-time jobs or, for those who are unable to work, supervised recreational activities and classes.

full-time job in March 1993. It was then that I created the statewide self-advocacy group "Speaking for Ourselves." I was able to help people from around the state speak up for what they wanted and needed to make their lives as meaningful as possible. In November 1993, I coordinated the first "Speaking for Ourselves" conference. That was the first time there had ever been a conference in Maine for people with developmental disabilities. In 1993, 300 people attended; in 1994, 400; and in 1995 there were 450.

In the course of my career I have also helped those people with special needs get involved with speaking before legislators and other influential people about issues, such as funding for various programs, that affect them. It is really neat to be able to help people speak for the first time and watch the reaction they get. It gives them a sense of knowing they can make a difference; their voices are being heard and others are listening.

Community Support Services has helped many people, including myself, to become more independent. I would like to share a few of their success stories.

Sandra was living in one of the Medicaid waiver homes run by CSSI that provides staffing around the clock. She wanted to move into her own apartment, but because she had epilepsy, her family was very much against the idea of her moving into a place by herself. With my help, Sandra convinced everyone that she was capable of living on her own, and in March 1994 she finally moved into her own apartment. In the beginning she was getting support forty hours a week, learning how to cook and perform other daily living skills and receiving transportation to appointments, but this was soon reduced to between five and ten hours a week. Sandra became very involved with both the local and state self-advocacy groups and was on the board of directors for a support services group.

Sandra underwent brain surgery in October 1996 to try to control the seizures she had been experiencing and suffered a stroke on the left side of her brain. She died on October 13. The last words she spoke before entering a coma were these: "I have achieved everything I wanted in life. I wanted to live in my own apartment and I did."

Linda, who has cerebral palsy, is another person who has been helped by CSSI. She was living in a four-person Medicaid waiver home, but wanted to move into an apartment with just one roommate. Linda advocated for herself and kept telling everyone what she wanted. She even spoke to the commissioner of the Department of Mental Health/Mental Retardation to prove she was capable of leaving the home. It took a long time and Linda got very frustrated during the process, but finally, in January 1996, she moved into her own apartment with a roommate. She is now able to hire her own staff and is more independent. She has twenty-four-hour staffing because both she and her roommate are in wheelchairs. The apartment is very close to where she attends day programming. Recently, Linda went to Walt Disney World on a vacation!

CSSI provides whatever services people need to be able to live their lives as independently as possible. Sandra and Linda are just two of the many stories I could share with you. It makes me feel that my job is worthwhile when I can help people fulfill their dreams of living more independently.

I recently changed jobs and I am currently working for the State of Maine in the the office of Consumer Affairs for the Department of Mental Health, Mental Retardation, and Substance Abuse Services. I'm the consumer advocate for people with developmental disabilities. Our office is staffed with four people, all of whom have disabilities. We are the first state in the nation to have an office where people with cross-disabilities are working together. I'm also starting to write a book about my experiences.

I have received a number of awards, including the Victory Award for Maine. This award is given by the governor of each state to individuals who have overcome obstacles. All the winners attend a ceremony at the JFK Center in Washington, D.C. In January 1988, I was a guest on the Christian Broadcasting Network's "700 Club" and in May 1996, I was featured on the "Today" show. I have also been written up in *Psychology Today* and *Hope* magazines.

Some personal goals that I have achieved include graduating from the University of Maine at Farmington and the work I did as the self-advocacy organizer for CSSI. Living independently in my own apartment is very important to me. I feel good about working to change the way people feel about and treat people with disabilities. If I could change one thing in my life, I would like to be able to live a normal life without pain or having to wear hearing aides, glasses, or high-top shoes all the time. Also, I would like to be free of taking medications.

The thing that I value most is that I am still alive. I am forty-four and can still work and do most things for myself without assistance. Having a disability has given me a special appreciation for things. I value spending time with my friends and family and time is precious to me. None of us knows how long we will be here, so I value each day and live it to the fullest.

My plans for the future include finding a way to make enough money to live my life without having to worry about how to support myself. Someday I hope to find the right person with whom to share my life and get married. If I had one message to communicate to others, it would be to take a hard look at the word "disability," because within that word is the word "ability."

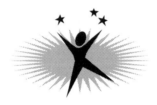

Undercover Angel:
A Guardian for Our Youth

Patrick Walsh

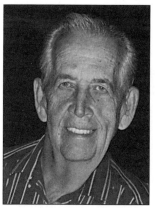

Patrick Walsh, now in his mid-sixties, was diagnosed with cerebral palsy at the age of six. He volunteered twelve years of his life as an undercover drug enforcement officer and has been credited with keeping substantial quantities of heroin and other narcotics from entering the United States. He spent four years volunteering for the Phoenix chapter of the Guardian Angels and was a member of his local Neighbors on Patrol group, where he patrolled downtown Phoenix monitoring and reporting drug sites and crack houses to the police.

It was not until I was six that my cerebral palsy was correctly diagnosed. Prior to that the doctors that examined me assumed that I had infantile paralysis (polio). In my case, the cerebral palsy was probably caused by spinal nerve injury at birth possibly due to my large size—I weighed ten and a half pounds! Even now, at the age of sixty-six, I hesitate to use the term "disability" or "handicap" to describe my condition. Long ago I realized that "disability" or "handicap" is the appropriate word only if you let your condition overcome your abilities.

*Editor's note: Some names in this chapter have been changed to protect the privacy of those involved.

Until I reached the age of eight I had very limited ability to walk or sit up without additional support, but I realized early on that my cerebral palsy would be considered moderate compared to many others who required constant, life-long care.

Because of the damage to the nerves in my spine, cerebral palsy causes a constriction of the tendons in both my legs, my groin, and to a lesser degree, in my arms. When I was eight two doctors suggested to my mother that I might benefit from an experimental operation that would become known as tendon ligation. After implanting animal tendons (I believe they were from a goat) in both ankles and on both sides of my groin, I was able to stand alone and walk normally without stumbling and falling. Lengthening my tendons with the animal implants allowed me more movement in my legs, which in turn provided me better balance while walking, although I still have a rather awkward gait. At last I could do things that my brother was able to do: walk to the store by myself, climb stairs, and ride a tricycle.

In 1943, when I was fourteen, I had a second tendon ligation operation to lengthen the tendons behind my knees, which improved my standing posture. Due to my operations, however, I did not graduate from high school until I was eighteen.

By attending classes nights and vacations during my last three years in high school, I earned a degree in accounting from a local business college in 1947, at the same time I received my high school diploma. I found that I had a gift of the "Irish Blarney"—I could talk a blue streak— and spent most of my adult working years in sales. After a few years in book and magazine sales, I became interested in photography, which lead to thirty years in various facets in photography sales and promotion.

In 1969, when I was forty, I was working with a transient (town-to-town) portrait photographer and we were setting up to work in Nogales, Arizona, which is on the Mexican border about two hundred miles south of Phoenix. One night while I was enjoying a cold beer and a floor show in Sonora, Mexico, a man asked me if I knew someone in Phoenix who might want to buy quantities of heroin. I was not a prude or naive but I was in total shock that he would even ask me. I quickly recovered and replied that I might be interested if the price was right and no risk would be involved. How little did Roberto Diaz know that I intended to relay his offer to the first law enforcement agency (on the U.S. side of the border) that I could contact the next morning.

I reasoned that if I could stop just one dirt bag (now a favorite name for anyone dealing with drugs) I could possibly stop drugs from reaching my seventeen-year-old son whom I had not seen since his mother and I divorced sixteen years previously when he and his sister were both very young children.

The next day I contacted the U.S. Customs Agency Service in Nogales and was introduced to narcotics agent Horace Cavitt. The authorities were interested in doing business with Diaz, whom, I learned later, had a long history of cross-border drug dealings. Horace recruited me as a volunteer informant and cautioned me about the pitfalls and dangers that might be involved. He encouraged me to move to the Mexican side of the border on the chance that I might be able to identify other customers and acquaintances of Diaz. I moved into the Alhambra hotel that day and was immediately accepted into the confidences of several locals. Some warned me to stay away from Roberto Diaz and tried to steer me to other drug sources.

Inasmuch as my high school Spanish had improved to the degree of passable "border" Spanish, I could converse and understand most conversations. Usually when I was introduced, the phrase "bueno gente" was added, meaning that I was "good people and could be trusted."

After I was at the Alhambra for about a week, Diaz approached me with some urgency. He had a friend who wanted to move large amounts of marijuana cheaply and in a hurry. I said that I would have to contact my friend in Phoenix first and that I would let him know something later that same day.

I immediately contacted Agent Cavitt and filled him in. He requested that I locate where the marijuana was stored on the pretense of setting up a buy for six hundred pounds of marijuana.

Over a beer in a Santana bar, about seventy miles south of the Arizona/Sonora Border, I told the wholesaler, Jesus Sepulveda, that my buyer in Phoenix had to be convinced that six hundred pounds of "*mota*" would be waiting when he flew down and that the price would be a firm $30 per pound. Sepulveda assured me the price was firm and to prove that he had the large amount available we would have to take a ride outside of town to his ranch.

He refused to let Roberto Diaz go along to the ranch because Sepulveda did not trust him—Diaz had supposedly ripped him off previously.

With Sepulveda's bodyguard driving my car we drove west for about seven miles. We turned left onto a dirt ranch road and proceeded about three-quarters of a mile and stopped. The driver turned the car's headlights on and off three times and then we proceeded past an adobe house for about another quarter mile and stopped. It didn't dawn on me until later the business with the headlights was a signal to guards in the house.

We soon arrived at a gate, got out of the car, and walked a short distance through a second gate. We stopped near a cluster of small trees.

Sepulveda's bodyguard began removing damp sand that was laying over a canvas. The canvas was pulled back and row after row of "kilo bricks" of marijuana were exposed.

Sepulveda reached down and picked up a "brick" and broke it open for me to examine. To prove that I wasn't ignorant, I smelled it and felt to see how dry it was. Sepulveda assured me that the marijuana was mature and had nice long "fingers." (The length of the leaves, "fingers," indicate how mature the marijuana is.)

After the "cache" was properly covered again, Sepulveda seemed to want to hang around and talk. He inquired about my handicap (by that time I was walking with a cane), my profession, and how long I had known Diaz. Apparently, even in my border Spanish, my answers convinced Sepulveda that I was a truly *"muy bueno gente"* and that we could do business.

Diaz and I drove back to Nogales, Sonora,* arriving there at about 3:00 A.M. I dropped him off at his house and immediately crossed over to the Arizona side of the border and phoned Horace Cavitt.

Horace and I met at a restaurant and went into the closed dining room where I drew a detailed map showing where Sepulveda had his "cache" of marijuana buried. I then returned to the Alhambra Hotel on the Mexican side of the border and slept nervously until

---

*There are towns by the name of Nogales on both the Mexican and American sides of the border.

early evening. What I didn't know was that while I slept the Mexican Federal Police and two U.S. Customs undercover agents used my map to seize over 1,500 kilograms (well over 3,000 pounds) of marijuana from the ranch of Jesus Sepulveda. They arrested Sepulveda and his bodyguard. Sepulveda was later convicted and spent four months in jail before becoming an informant for the U.S. Customs Department.

The Sepulveda incident was probably the largest, most satisfying seizure that I arranged during my twelve years as a volunteer informant for U.S. Customs Agency Service and Drug Enforcement Administration.

There was only one time in my career as an informant that I felt that my life was possibly in danger. There was a seizure involving forty ounces of heroin, in which I had convinced a man named Juan Menendez to deliver the heroin and cocaine to me on credit to the Arizona side of the border. His "mule," the person carrying the shipment, delivered it and was arrested. I never returned to Naco, Sonora, to pay Menendez for his drugs.

Having heard that Menendez was seriously ill with tuberculosis and would probably not recover, I was brave enough to return to a nearby border town (Agua Prieta, Sonora). While I was there Juan Menendez of Naco drove up to me and demanded the money that I owed him.

Again, my border Spanish saved my life. I was able to convince Menendez that I had been burnt (turned in by his "mule") and had only recently got out of prison. I told Menendez that I would return to Naco the following weekend and pay him $500 a week until I had paid him the thousands of dollars that I owed him. I can only guess that his stupidity and greed allowed me to walk away that day, never to return to Naco or Agua Prieta again.

I have never let being an informant, snitch, or "finger" bother me. I believe that by keeping any amount of dangerous drugs off the streets and out of schools I might save the life of one person.

In 1982, I decided that I could no longer expend the energy or my financial resources to continue my desire to keep drugs off the streets and out of the hands of innocent children. I decided to slow down and simply try to support myself to the best of my ability. My cerebral palsy wasn't getting worse (cerebral palsy is not a degenerative condition), but age and encroaching problems with arthritis were beginning to take their toll on my body.

In my twelve years as an informant with the U.S. Customs Agency service and the U.S. Drug Administration I was paid approximately $1,200, and in most cases I did not recoup my out-of-pocket expenses. Even so, I have absolutely no regrets, as I view my efforts as a labor of love. I think that my disability was a good disguise in my undercover efforts, because no one believed that someone with cerebral palsy would ever volunteer for such a physically and emotionally demanding effort.

In 1989, Curtis Sliwa, the founder of the Guardian Angels, a group of volunteers dedicated to preventing crime through example and deeds, came to Phoenix to organize a local chapter. I had heard of their anti-drug/crime fighting efforts in other cities and I believed (and still believe) that the Guardian Angels Program is the most effective anticrime effort ever devised for volunteers who want to make a difference. I had originally intended to pay a courtesy visit to their headquarters and welcome them to the Phoenix area, but I got caught up in their youthful enthusiasm and, at the age of sixty-six, became the first senior citizen member in the Phoenix chapter.

I was not physically able to participate in neighborhood foot patrols, but I practically wore out my old Chevette conducting mobile patrols to warn those on foot of possible trouble spots ahead.

Our first year's efforts paid off in the closure of the El Rancho Motel and the 902 Bar, two very high-profile locations for prostitution and drug sales. My most gratifying experiences were visiting schools and talking to students about the dangers of drugs and street gangs.

I was able to spend a very satisfying four years with the Guardian Angels, until April 1993; and I spent the last fifteen months as chapter leader.

For the past two and a half years I have been involved with a group of older concerned citizens. Our "Neighbors on Patrol" targets two of the highest crime neighborhoods in the city of Phoenix. We patrol at least two nights every week targeting crack houses and areas of curb-side drug sales and prostitution. We monitor known drug sites and prepare regular reports and turn them over to the Phoenix police department. I also became involved in a program in which the Oakland/University Park Neighborhood Association prosecutes landlords that continue to rent to crack dealers after our patrol establishes a pattern of abuse. The association received the 1996 Mayor's Award as the most outstanding neighborhood association in the city of Phoenix. Shortly afterward I had to resign from Neighbors on Patrol because of increasing problems with arthritis, but I am confident someone will take my place.

If I could change one thing in my life, it would be to have had the opportunity to watch my son and daughter grow into adulthood. I have, however, been able to renew my association with my son and daughter, and thus I now derive some consolation by watching my three grandsons and one granddaughter grow up.

Over the years I have been fortunate to work with many dedicated drug enforcement agents who accepted my volunteer efforts at face value, although a few questioned my motivation, considering my apparent physical limitations. My response to them was that maybe because of my limited physical abilities I would be able to infiltrate unsuspecting areas of the drug underworld.

I would urge anyone who reads this to get involved in Neighbors on Patrol or help organize a similar program so that our young people can have a chance to grow up in a drug- and gang-free society.

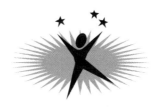

More Than an Average Guy

Larry Patton

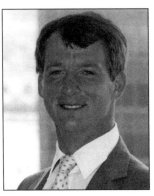

Larry Patton was diagnosed with cerebral palsy due to complications at birth. While working for IBM, he developed People Helping People through Technology, a marketing program for IBM's technology for the disabled that helps companies better understand the barriers that limit the disabled in the workforce. He currently works for TECH 2000: Michigan's Assistive Technology Project as a development specialist.

I have faced many hurdles and obstacles throughout my life. I hope that you find encouragement and strength from my story. My first hurdle began at birth. During my delivery the umbilical cord was wrapped tightly around my neck, and I had to wait twenty-five minutes until I could take my first breath of air. The cord was so tightly tangled that the marks it left on my neck were visible for several months. As a result of my not breathing, my brain did not receive oxygen and at the age of two I was diagnosed with cerebral palsy. Although in my case the culprit was lack of oxygen, cerebral palsy (CP) can be caused by any type of damage to the brain that results in a loss of brain cells. The condition prevents those who have it from controlling parts of their body because the connections between the involved sections of the brain are incomplete. There are varying degrees of CP: some people use wheelchairs or are unable to speak while others may only have a slight limp when they walk. Cerebral palsy is not curable, but it does not get worse as time passes. In my case, CP affects only my fine motor skills, which means I cannot do anything that requires manual dexterity.

One of the motor skills that is affected is my speech. Many people have trouble understanding what I am saying when they talk to me for the first time. I also have difficulty walking—I can wear out a pair of shoes in three to five months. I have two different size feet and always have to buy two pairs of shoes. In addition to having difficulty speaking and walking, it is hard or almost impossible for me to manage buttons, tie shoes, or to thread a needle, and I cannot write legibly. It is a common misconception that people with cerebral palsy are also mentally impaired. The fact is, however, the cerebral palsy only affects my motor skills and does not affect any part of my mind.

My parents played a very important role in shaping who I am today. My mother never allowed me to see any of her frustration or discouragement in dealing with my handicap. My father had a quiet and gentle spirit, and spent a lot of quality time with my brother and me.

My parents treated my brother and me equally while we were growing up. I was expected to do my share of chores. My parents' philosophy was that I should try everything at least once and if I couldn't do it then we would try to find an alternative way of doing it. This applied to daily functions such as feeding and dressing myself, as well as other skills, such as riding a bike, walking, and other activities.

My Christian upbringing and active membership in

our church became very important factors in my life. My family and church accepted me unconditionally despite my physical condition—they did not see the handicap. Over the years, I have learned that my friends, too, do not see me as disabled.

While growing up, I was included in social functions in the neighborhood, at school, and at church. Despite the fact that my friends and family accepted me, the biggest hurdle that I have faced in my life has been accepting myself for who I am. It was very difficult and depressing at times to look at myself in a mirror because I would be reminded of who I thought I really was: An individual with an obvious disability. It was especially hard when I reached the age where I began dating girls. I would ask women to go out on a date to see a movie or maybe go to dinner and nine times out of ten they would reject my invitation.

When the invitation was accepted and I did go on a date I would have a great time and get the impression that the young lady whom I was with was also having a good time. But by the third or fourth date, I always heard the same message in different words: "Larry, you are a great guy, but I do not want to go out with you anymore," "Larry, I do not want to get serious with you," or "I like you and I want to be your friend but I am not interested in starting a romantic relationship with you." I could not understand why these women wanted to be my friend but were not interested in dating me. For me, the answer was my handicap. The more rejection I received from women, the harder it was to accept myself. My greatest desire was to be loved by someone and, over time, it became harder to love myself. I found it difficult to understand why God had created me. I had to deal with the anger and frustration of not knowing why God allowed me to be handicapped. Even though I had been a Christian for many years I was still not able to look myself in the mirror and say, "I love you, Larry Patton."

This began to change when a major event took place in my life in November 1984. I asked a friend to pray with me for a physical healing of my cerebral palsy. I was on a tour of the Holy Land and we were sitting on the seashore of the Sea of Galilee in Israel when I experienced a miracle. I didn't receive physical healing, but I began to accept myself for who I am. That day I began to fully understand that I am special.

It is interesting how fate works sometimes. Shortly after realizing that I am special, a young lady named Jennifer Ebaugh came into my life. I had made a decision to stop putting so much effort into dating because I believed God now fulfilled my desire to be loved. Because of this, I could be myself and I did not have to feel like I was performing or being someone I wasn't when I went out on dates. Probably for the first time in my life I was not trying to impress a woman. As a result of my new attitude toward dating, Jennifer and I simply became good friends.

Jenny and I met each other at a Christian young adults group that met once a week at her church. Jenny was raised a Catholic and I am a member of Protestant church. My church did not have any organized activities or fellowship groups for post-college-age individuals. Therefore, a friend of mine informed me about the young adults group and thought I would enjoy it. I began to enjoy Jenny's company and we started to do things together like going to dinner and to the movies. We spent many hours getting to know one another as friends.

There were three embarrassing moments that occurred between Jenny and me after we first became friends. The first occurred one weekend when most of the members from the group were away attending a conference and I asked Jenny if she would like to watch a movie on Friday evening. After the movie, Jenny and I were enjoying a pizza when I told her that I didn't know why I was hanging out with a group of Catholics because I could never marry one. Bad impression number one. The second incident occurred at an amusement park. We had enjoyed a great day together and it was time to begin thinking about starting the trip home. At that moment, I reached into my pocket and realized that my key ring was not there. My car, house, and office keys had more than likely come sliding out of my pocket on one of the roller coasters that afternoon. The trip home normally took an hour. On that summer evening it took us close to five hours to walk home. The final incident occurred later the same summer when I called Jenny's younger sister on the phone and asked her if she would accompany me to a friend's wedding. We had gone out as friends several times before I met Jenny, but this time she refused my invitation. I waited four to five minutes and proceeded to place another call to the same phone number. I was lucky because this time Jenny answered the phone. I extended the same invitation to her and she accepted. I asked her if she could meet me at my house. I was an hour late meeting Jenny for the wedding because I was stuck in the middle of a golf tournament. All I can figure is that Jenny and I were meant to be together.

By getting past and laughing about these rather embarrassing moments, we established a very deep and close friendship before we decided to start seeing each other on a romantic basis. The first thing that attracted me to her as a friend was her openness to my physical handicap. She was able to look beyond it and get to know the real Larry Patton.

Jenny's faith; her caring nature for others, especially children; and her loving, gentle spirit were all qualities that led me to ask her to be my wife. On June 12, 1987, we were married. It was the single happiest day of my life.

In 1990, I was working as a systems engineer in the marketing division of IBM. The best way to describe my job is that I helped my customers with the design, development, installation, and support of computer hardware and software packages and applications. One day a customer came to me with a question that ended up having a major impact on my career. The customer had worked for an automobile company for over twenty-five years and was having a problem seeing his computer screen. He had his eyes checked and it was determined that he had a degenerative visual impairment. Now, in order to read his computer display, he had to place his nose on the screen. He wanted to know if IBM had any products that could assist him with reading his computer screen.

After a week of research, I was able to find a much larger computer display for my customer, who was very satisfied with the solution. Even so, I was concerned because this customer did not feel comfortable voicing his problem to his management team. Even though he had been with his company more than twenty-five years, he felt that he might be discriminated against if he made it known that he was losing his eyesight. Over the next several days, his problem kept entering my thoughts.

During lunch one day, I relayed this experience to my manager, and in the course of our conversation, I wondered aloud how many other customers with unseen or seen disabilities might be more productive using the right technology. As a result of this discussion, I was asked to develop a business plan for implementing a program that would address the technology needs of our customers with disabilities. After six months of research and development, my business plan was accepted by IBM and the People Helping People through Technology program began in Detroit.

The Americans with Disabilities Act (ADA), which extends federal civil rights laws to protect people with disabilities from job discrimination, had just been passed by Congress. Under the act, employers with more than fifteen employees cannot deny employment to a person with a disability who has the qualifications for the job. The ADA requires employers to make reasonable accommodation for a qualified individual with a known physical or mental disability. Potential reasonable accommodations might include job restructuring, reassignment to a vacant position, part-time or modified work schedules, assistive technology devices or services, or qualified interpreters.

Every day we take a lot for granted. Most of us have no difficulty opening a door, turning on a light switch, taking a pen out of a pocket, using a personal computer, answering a phone, or reading a newspaper, but more than 43 million Americans cannot perform one or more of these functions without the help of a personal assistant or the aid of technology. People Helping People through Technology was a program to introduce our customers to computer-related technology that could provide reasonable accommodations to people with disabilities in their work environment.

Assistive technology is defined as any item, piece of equipment, or product system that is used to increase, maintain, or improve functional capabilities of individuals with disabilities. We are surrounded by, and take for granted, many kinds of technology—telephones, VCRs, personal computers, and fax machines, to name a few. Assistive technology is becoming nearly as common and important in the lives of people with disabilities. This technology includes all the tools, both high- and low-tech, that people with disabilities can use to make their lives more independent and fulfilling.

Computer technology, one form of assistive technology, has enormous potential to improve the lives of people with disabilities. Computers can provide a voice to persons who cannot speak; permit written communication to persons with fine motor impairments and learning disabilities; allow telephone communication between persons with hearing impairments; encourage reading by persons with visual impairments; permit and improve the productive employment capability of adults with disabilities; and support and improve the ability of persons with disabilities to live as independently as possible.

The major activities of the People Helping People through Technology program were executive awareness presentations, assistive technology demonstrations, educational assistance, and customer support assistance. The program educated individuals about the barriers that limit people with disabilities in the workforce, explained ways to comply with Americans with Disabilities Act, and exposed individuals to assistive technology devices like the IBM Independence series of products, which include speech recognition programs, text-to-speech conversion tools, and telephone communication systems.

For the two and a half years that the People Helping People through Technology program existed, I had a demonstration facility at IBM which featured different types of assistive technology. This center was used to educate business executives on the different types of technology and software applications available to assist individuals with disabilities. In creating the demonstration center, I was able to develop a partnership with a local company, ComputAbility, which specialized in providing assistive technology for personal computers, allowing individuals with mobility, vision, or hearing impairments to use personal computers. ComputAbility placed their technology devices and products in our demonstration center, complementing the IBM products. The partnership was very successful and we were able to show a total solution for individuals with disabilities in both employment and education settings.

These solutions included different types of computer technology and software that were designed to increase one's productivity on the job and in many cases made it possible for individuals with disabilities to obtain employment. I also hosted presentations in the evening for educators and parents of children with disabilities. It was very rewarding when someone came to a presentation or demonstration and said "I have an employee" or "I have a friend who could benefit from using this assistive technology device." The People Helping People through Technology program was the highlight of my sixteen-year IBM career because I was able to assist individuals with disabilities to lead more productive lives.

Early in March 1993, two days after I received the "Disabled Computer Scientist Employee of the Year" award in Washington, D.C., I was told by my manager at IBM that as of June 30 I would no longer have a job with IBM, which was going through a major downsizing effort. The People Helping People through Technology program could have been labeled as a good public relations campaign or a good community project, but the program did not pay for itself because we were not selling enough hardware and software. I was one of 100,000 employees affected by layoffs.

Jenny returned to teaching and was able to get her old job back teaching third grade to compensate for our reduced income. She learned how to manage her time being a wife, mother to the son we had adopted in 1991, and teacher, and I became Mr. Mom, which proved to be very rewarding. Our son, William, had just turned two years old and during the day I learned to dress him, provide meals, and meet his daily needs. It was another learning opportunity for me.

On December 8, 1993, less than six months after leaving IBM, my prayers were answered and I found a new job. I accepted a position with the State of Michigan working on the TECH 2000: Michigan's Assistive Technology Project.

The mission of TECH 2000 is to increase funding and access to assistive technology by developing linkages that create a statewide system change and advocacy network that is consumer driven, community based, and permanent. System change is a change in law or policy at a local, state, or federal level that is permanent and affects all individuals in similar situations. It does not apply to just one individual or one family, and it is not temporary. The change in policy and practices permanently improves access to assistive technology services and devices.

While skiing last winter in the Colorado Rockies, I thought about what it must have been like for the American pioneers in the late 1800s to cross over these mountains. They probably encountered many difficult challenges, obstacles, and barriers while carving a new pathway through the great frontier. The pioneers were individuals with dreams. To make their dreams become reality they had to be able to visualize them and be willing to take risks. The American pioneers had no guarantee that their new journey would work because they had very little experience. They acted on faith and intuition with a lot of excitement and enthusiasm. The TECH 2000 project is like the American pioneer blazing new trails by providing new solutions and avenues for accessing assistive technology to consumers, parents, employers, and others throughout the state of Michigan. If we achieve the desired outcome it will mean equal opportunity for everyone at school, on the job, at home, or while enjoying recreational activities.

Individuals with disabilities have been brainwashed into believing that they should settle for less. I am here to say that if you have a dream or vision, do not settle for anything less than achieving your goal. Do not allow people to stop you from being all you can or want to be. Only you can decide if you are going to be a pioneer.

I have always lived my life as a pioneer, helping others to achieve their dreams. In 1981, my mother and I started an eight-year project of gathering information to write my biography. The book, *More Than an Average Guy,* was released about ten years ago.* This book shares how I have overcome the same things most people take for granted. With each new obstacle or hurdle that I face in life, I try to always persevere with courage and motivation.

More Than An Average Guy is not just an inspirational biography of a disabled boy; it is the story of a family raising a disabled child. The narrative is told from

---

*Janet Krastner, *More Than an Average Guy: The Story of Larry Patton* (Canton, Ohio: Life Enrichment Publishers, 1989).

several viewpoints: my parents', my younger brother's, my grandparents', and friends' and neighbors'. All explain how they were affected by my cerebral palsy.

In 1985 I founded the Hurdling Handicaps Speaking Ministry. This is a Christ-centered ministry for people to see and hear how God works in extraordinary and powerful ways to overcome life's challenges. Hurdling Handicaps has taken me across the United States sharing my story, encouraging others to hurdle the handicaps of life, whatever they may be, physical, emotional, or spiritual. I believe that we all have some kind of handicap to overcome. The only difference is that you can see mine.

I have found that life is not always fair. Many people who face obstacles and hurdles ask, "Why me?" I believe that everything happens for a reason. Even though I have experienced many obstacles and disappointments, I have also been blessed with a beautiful family and a rewarding career helping people. There will always be obstacles, but if you persevere you will always be able to achieve your goals.

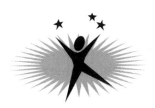

Dare to Dream:
Finding Ability in Disability

Marcia Boehm

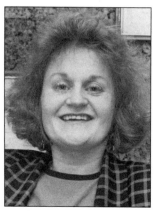

Marcia Boehm, a social worker currently working toward her doctorate in adult education, was born with over twenty-five multiple fractures due to osteogenesis imperfecta, otherwise known as brittle bone disorder. She is president and CEO of Person Ability, a nonprofit organization that focuses on maximizing individual and organizational potential by providing consulting services to businesses and nursing homes; divorce and school mediation; and counseling to people with disabilities, the elderly, and other minority groups.

The day I was born was a beautiful day full of anticipation and excitement. My mom gave birth to her first baby girl. It was then when she discovered that I, her new baby, was born with multiple bone fractures. It had been a hard labor, but there were no explanations for what had occurred. Everything about me seemed normal except for multiple fractures at twenty-five different sites in my body. The doctors weren't sure if I would live, but they told my mother that if I survived the next three days I would be fine. The doctors knew very little about my condition, osteogenesis imperfecta, often referred to as "the brittle bone disorder."

118

Osteogenesis imperfecta (OI) is a genetic disorder characterized by bones that break easily, often from little or no apparent cause. There are at least four distinct forms of the disorder representing extreme variation in severity from one individual to another. A person may have as few as ten or as many as several hundred fractures in a lifetime. While the number of persons affected with OI in the United States is unknown, the best estimate suggests there may be as many as 50,000 cases. Most forms of OI are caused by imperfectly formed bone collagen resulting from a genetic defect. Collagen is the major protein of the body's connective tissue and can be likened to the framework around which a building is constructed. In cases of OI a person has either less or a poorer quality of collagen. The characteristic features of OI vary greatly from person to person and not all characteristics are evident in each case.

Once I was released from the hospital three weeks after I was born, my mom had to carry me around on a pillow because of the fragility of my bones—even holding me in her arms could cause one or more to break. The doctors informed her that I would never walk or live what others called a "normal life" due to the nature of my problem. My bones would curve and fracture as I grew. A surgical technique of breaking and resetting bones in order to straighten and thereby strengthen them was available, but at first the doctors would not perform it on me. When I was five years old, however, I went to Children's Hospital in Detroit for what were supposed to be routine X-rays. Instead of the usual information, though, this set of X-rays revealed ball sockets that had never shown up before (not everyone is born with ball sockets and previously the doctors had never seen any in my X-rays). These ball sockets would finally allow the doctors to perform the surgery.

This began a series of multiple hospital visits and numerous surgeries, most of which occurred when I was between the ages of five and fifteen. I had had more than twenty-five surgeries by the time I turned fifteen, many of which included inserting rush rods into the femur and tibia bones in my legs. The rods reduced the number of future surgeries that I would need because they protected my bones from additional curving, but I can never forget the instability of my bones.

During my most recent fracture, my doctors discovered I not only had a broken bone, but also a broken steel rush rod. According to my doctor this was a very unusual situation for someone with my bone condition. His hope was to try to replace the old rod with a new one, in the least invasive way. He wanted to interact with my bone on a very minimal basis because of its fragility. Too much or too forceful interaction could do more damage than good to the bone. A term currently used to describe the nature of my bone is "peanut brittle"—it's hard, but it can shatter. During the surgery, which was scheduled for right after the first of the year, I experienced complications. The doctor wasn't able to remove the whole rod but only a portion of it because of the location and angle of the surgical site and his concern about being to invasive. I experienced respiratory difficulties due to asthma (with which I had been diagnosed at age seven) and the stress of the situation. I was sent home from the hospital to see a trauma specialist, a consultation that brought about a plan of action calling for surgical intervention from the knee up to remove the rest of the old rod and replace it with a one made of titanium, a metal much stronger than steel. The specialist added three screws to the rod to further ensure that it would not move, giving it greater stability.

The characteristics of titanium also give it more bend, which was important given the bend in my bones. I am now finally on the road to recovery, but it has been a difficult process. I was in two different hospitals within a month for almost three weeks total, and due to the lack of experience of the medical profession with OI, many have not learned to listen to the patient.

It's funny, people often think that the more surgeries you have, the easier it is to deal with the stress of surgery; that somehow you get "used" to it. In fact, I believe it's quite the opposite. You become more aware of your mortality. I suppose that working in a hospital for so many years (I had worked as a social worker in hospitals ever since I completed my bachelor's degree) makes me even more aware of what can go wrong. When I was twenty years old I was in a car accident and broke my arm. Soon afterward I began experiencing severe back pain. As a result of the pain, I was diagnosed with scoliosis, curvature of the spine. I was shocked when I heard the diagnosis. No one had ever told me that I had this condition and I had been seen by some of the best doctors. I was told that if I didn't undergo a spinal fusion, a process that permanently joins two or more vertebrae to strengthen or straighten them, I would have increased difficulty with my breathing. (The hunched posture that results from scoliosis reduces the space available in the chest cavity, squeezing the lungs and making it difficult for them to expand when breathing.) I remember being told that there was a chance that I could become paralyzed because of the surgery, but not having the surgery could have resulted in other problems later in my life. I was devastated because I had finally begun to be independent. I had broken up with my fiancé and found a new boyfriend who later became my husband. I was working, had a car, and was frequently out with my friends. It didn't seem fair. Because the surgery would require me to be in a body cast for one year, I would have to move back home and have others help me during my recovery. I remember thinking it had been easier when I was younger because my mom made the decisions—it wasn't up to me. Now I had to make the decisions. After a lot of thought, I decided to have the surgery. I remember trying to break up with David, my boyfriend, before the surgery was performed because I didn't want him to feel obligated to be with me. I told him I didn't think our relationship was working out and that I didn't want to see him anymore. He of course figured it out and assured me he was there because he wanted to be, not because he felt he had to be.

After I had the surgery I woke up with a tube down my throat, but I didn't realize it was there because I couldn't see it. I thought I was paralyzed in my mouth and I wouldn't be able to talk. I was petrified. I was young and impressionable. I remember thinking that Mama Cass of the group the Mamas and the Papas had recently died by choking on a ham sandwich and that I was going to die too. My mom and David weren't there when I woke up, which increased my fear. I wondered if I had already died. I wasn't sure where I was and it was a big room. I didn't know I was in intensive care, nor did I know that there were limited hours for family/friends to be in the room with you. I was also unaware I was only in a half-body cast; that the rest of the cast would be put on after the swelling in my back had subsided. I remember that when my mom and David finally came in to see me I was very relieved. I wanted to tell them I was going to die, so they would be ready; I didn't want it to be a surprise to them. I tried to write it in the air and they thought I was telling them I loved them. Later that day, in front of me, the doctors argued about whether I could come off the respirator. I was frightened and filled with so many different emotions—what if they took me off the respirator but the doctor who had argued that I was ready was wrong? I still remember those feelings clearly, and every time I have surgery they are resurrected.

My last surgery was no different; it triggered some of those same emotions. Now, a year later, I am still not completely healed. I have begun visualization techniques to help with the healing process. Mentally, I picture the bones healing and becoming stronger, and this helps me cope with the slow process of becoming whole. It has been a year now and the pain is not as acute; however, I am always reminded that I can't take life for granted. There are times when the pain is greater: if I'm tired or if the weather is cold or humid. I can tell when I'm overly stressed because my leg or my back give me more pain than on a normal day.

I believe this experience has reinforced my personal philosophy that disabilities are not an oddity in one's life, but just a part of the continuum of life. If people live long enough they will encounter issues related to disabilities within their own life.

For a good portion of my life I remember thinking that my disability was just one of the inconveniences I would have to deal with. I sometimes tell people that I was too dumb to know that I was "different," that I was supposed to be less successful or less capable than someone healthy, and I never learned to live up to society's expectations. I was always rather friendly and learned at an early age how to connect with people. I think that social ability can be a greater gift than a high IQ.

Everyone has abilities and part of our life journey is

to discover them both in ourselves and others. As a child, I learned not to draw attention to my disability, but instead to assimilate into the able-bodied world. I remember telling a friend that when I went to college I didn't look for someone with a disability to be my mentor because I wanted to be successful. I now think that is a sad and tragic statement. I no longer see or believe that people with disabilities should assimilate into the able-bodied world. Architectural and environmental changes assist more than just people with disabilities. For example, curb cuts benefit wheelchair users as well as moms with strollers and people riding bikes. Handicap bathroom stalls assist the elderly and parents who need extra space to help their small children. If people live long enough they will encounter issues related to disabilities within their school, workplace, or community.

The removal of environmental barriers is an extremely important issue to those with disabilities, but the most difficult issue I have faced is dealing with people's attitudes and beliefs, which tend to reinforce negative stereotypes and myths about people with disabilities. I am certain that there are jobs I wasn't considered for because I didn't fit the interviewer's image of how an employee should look. I have been very fortunate and continued to persevere. I found many successes along my path of life. I have been categorized as "spunky," spirited, and enthusiastic. I think these qualities have enabled me to not take no for an answer. It has been my experience that not all discrimination in intentional. Able-bodied individuals sometimes don't know or understand the issues unless they are told about them. When I find people uncomfortable or lacking in knowledge about disabilities in general or my disability specifically, I help them gain a new perspective by using humor and by educating them.

I have been fortunate to have people in my life who believed in my ability to make the world a better place. I am very grateful to my mom, dad, stepdad, brother, grandparents, husband, and friends. I also had many mentors along the way who taught me things I needed to learn. My mom taught me discipline and was relentless in not treating me differently or giving me special breaks because I had a disability. In fact, she held me to a higher standard for which I am now deeply grateful. For example, she taught me that there was more than one way to be a dancer. One didn't always have to stand on her toes to dance. Dancing is more about an approach, a commitment to keep trying, even when we are tired. It's about creativity, sparkle, zest, and perseverance. I have learned to dance, see, experience, and feel the movement in and around me. My dad taught me about the gift of gab and how to connect with people. My younger brother, Rusty, was my rock, my protector, and my salvation as a child. When we were kids, we were best friends. I know I wouldn't be who I am today without him. Rose believed more in my ability to start my business than I believed in myself. John, my stepdad, taught me about dependability and loyalty. David, my husband, is my stabilizer in a crisis. He has always allowed me the freedom to explore who I am and he helps me to do the things that aren't always physically easy for me to do. He shares my dreams and desires. Without all these people, as well as my children, my husband's family, and all who have played a significant part in my life, I would not be the person I am today.

Even though I have been blessed with many wonderful people, life has not always been easy. The physical barriers have been easier to confront than the deeply rooted attitudinal barriers presented by much of society. We don't always think of people with disabilities as having a culture or a history, but we should. Disability is not a circumstance, but rather a part of who someone is. People with disabilities can now claim their disability with pride as part of their identity.

Five years ago, after more than fourteen years, I left my position in a major metropolitan hospital. During my tenure I received numerous awards and was promoted to the position of director of my department. I continuously received outstanding performance reviews. One day, however, I was confronted with a new boss who clearly had internalized feelings about people with disabilities. Out of an organization of 4,000 employees, I was the only one at the level of department head who had a visible disability. At the new boss's behest, my position was eliminated a few days prior to the implementation of the Americans with Disabilities Act. I will always carry the scars that this experience caused. The wounds healed, but not quickly. Today, five years later, the scars continue to shape my being, forcing me to think about who I am and what I am doing.

The loss of this position hit me harder than I would have expected: it allowed every negative message that I had ever heard about myself to be replayed. Those messages take on greater degrees of importance to people with disabilities than perhaps they do to able-bodied individuals. Generally, people with disabilities have heard repeatedly messages that tell them the things that they can't do and few that tell them what they can do. Despite my achievements and the support I have received, this experience continues to plague me from time to time. Fortunately, I have been blessed with many successes since then. I know I am competent, but I still struggle with the issues of honesty, integrity, respect, and trustworthiness. Watching individuals within an organization in which you believed create their own reality—which may stray from the truth of the situation—has been difficult. It's painful, hurtful, and most of all damaging. This employment situation opened my eyes to the need for people with disabilities to find new and creative ways to experience themselves in successful situations. I recall a discussion with a dear friend of mine when I was trying to decide whether to litigate or agree to a settlement with the hospital. We asked ourselves, "What would have happened if there had been no Martin Luther King Jr. or Rosa Parks?" We decided that we couldn't turn our back on people with disabilities. That day I made a commitment to make a difference and although the lawsuit is not yet settled, I can be confident that my actions may give others the courage to fight for their rights, whether they are disabled or not.

After leaving the hospital I continued to work part-time in private practice as a therapist and I began working in the disabled community. I worked for nine months part-time as a program administrator and then accepted a position as the chief operating officer of two local centers for independent living. I thought that people with disabilities all functioned like myself. I believed they learned to compensate and assimilate into society. I had always been my own advocate but never asked for any special accommodations because I believed I shouldn't draw attention to my disability if I wanted to keep my job. While working at the centers I met many wonderful people and became more aware of the growing needs in this community. People with disabilities and other disenfranchised populations needed to gain more control over their lives. They needed to be provided with role models, leadership development, and employment opportunities. I saw a passion in people that was contagious. I rethought what I wanted my contribution to the world to be. I met people who challenged me in new ways. I found mentors. I learned about the possibilities within an individual that can be discovered when we value one another.

I worked full time with the centers for independent living for one year and then decided to start my own company. I knew I needed to try to start my own company because there were so many needs of people with disabilities and other minority individuals that were not being met by existing organizations. I needed to try to create programs that would begin to address some of these unmet needs and bring to the forefront the public policy and empowerment issues that were not being adequately addressed. I needed to identify core values and create a mission statement for my company, Person Ability. Person Ability counsels schools, families, and individuals on disability issues. We provide job development, life skills, and entrepreneur and empowerment training and counseling to both individuals and families primarily from disenfranchised groups. We counsel and advise organizations about training programs, visualization skills, return-to-work programs, human resource development and technical assistance for disabled employees, policy and leadership development, diversity, and motivational speaking.

We have been very fortunate and have grown at a rapid pace. We are funded through fee-for-service programs and grants from the state of Michigan and Wayne State University. We offer an empowerment training program (ACTS, Actively Creating Tools for Success) to individuals in Wayne, Oakland, and Macomb counties. The program focuses on self-exploration, communication skills, increasing self-esteem, and risk-taking and its relationship to vocational outcomes. It also explores the meaning of works and helps individuals set goals and develop action plans. We are also involved in an innovative school-to-work program in Macomb County, Michigan. We work with high school juniors and seniors and college students with disabilities and train them to become peer mentors. We match them up with younger disabled students transitioning into high school. Adult businessmen and -women with disabilities assist us by meeting and speaking with the students and discussing their challenges and successes.

We work with the Michigan Jobs Coalition to help people with disabilities develop résumés, practice interview skills, gain the confidence to work, and provide information on social security. We serve as consumer consultants on the Developmental Disabilities evaluation project at Michigan State University and recently we received a three-year project to work with employers within the three county areas to increase awareness and knowledge about hiring people with disabilities.

One of the values that emerged when I created Person Ability was having a passion for your work. If you have passion, your efforts will reflect it. If you walk the path on which your heart takes you, making life not a task or a duty but an adventure, then you will feel very different about what you do. I have learned an amazing amount about people and relationships over the past few years. I discovered that our minds will find wonderful answers when we ask ourselves the right questions. If we really love what we do and feel a burning passion for our work, then every experience associated with it will be enriching and growth-producing. Everything we do is meant to teach us something. Mistakes and misjudgments are only forks in the road that provide opportunities to make new choices and see new ways of doing things. Our mistakes or growth opportunities become stepping stones and when we climb these steps together we support one another in seeking new relationships, new ways of defining success and developing deeper levels of understanding. It is important that the entire staff of Person Ability help one another maintain a passion for what we do.

I also value the creativity that individuals bring to situations. I think it is important that we be open, receptive, and unafraid to step outside of the box. There is always more than one way to view a situation. For example, when my son was four, he loved to go down to the basement to play. He would say "Let's go play in the wheelchair." He certainly didn't hold the same fears or trepidations that adults have when they think of using a wheelchair. He didn't see the wheelchair as a limitation, but simply as different. To him, the situation was not right or wrong, it was just different.

Sometimes it is important just to listen. We don't always have to be right and we don't always have to know the right answer. In listening to our own silent moments, we may hear that one song, poem, or phrase that reminds us that what is outside of us is also inside of each of us. We can become the guides and the directors of our own experiences. We have the ability to imagine or reimagine the world the way it can be. It's important that our team at Person Ability is permitted to try things out that may not always work. We need to continue to explore and see what does work, to experience or discover the pleasure of the unexpected and the unique. I believe that as we support one another, we support our own levels of creativity. Each individual is powerful, but when we join together our collective "we" becomes even more powerful.

A third important value is balance, especially as it relates to family, friends, spirituality, and work. Our life must find balance in both our conscious intentions and the subtle forces that sometimes guide us as we go. When individuals don't find balance their perceptions of the world can become skewed, inaccurate. There is no greater gift than to share our lives. We are our greatest asset and when we share a piece of ourselves, we have shared our most prized possession.

I always struggle to achieve balance in my life. If I don't spend time with family and friends my perceptions of the world become one-sided; I lack creativity and the ability to see things in new ways. My relationships with my family and friends help me to think about my work and the world in new and different ways. My work with people helps me to bring ideas, thoughts, and personal stories to my personal life that may impact how those with whom I interact see or think about things. Everything in the world is interconnected; however, the ability to stay refreshed and energized is enhanced by our ability to find balance between our personal and professional life. When we don't find this balance we not only have a skewed perspective of the world but we can become resentful, angry, and ultimately sick. I remember reading in Dawna Markova's book *No Enemies Within** that illness or sickness is the Westerner's answer to meditation. It forces us

---

*Dawna Markova, *No Enemies Within: A Creative Process for Discovering What's Right about What's Wrong* (Berkeley, Calif.: Conari Press, 1994).

to take some time out. It becomes our approved way to think, listen, and reflect on where we are in our lives, allowing us to ask ourselves if our lives are balanced.

I highly value the ability to laugh at oneself. I think it important that we learn to live in the moment and not always take ourselves too seriously. We all experience things that create extra challenges or difficulties, but we can all overcome these obstacles. It is up to each individual. Some need more support than others, but each has the capacity to discover his or her own uniqueness, gifts, and talents. According to one definition, the word "crisis" means a time to decide. We need to remember, especially in times of crisis, that we have the ability to decide. On a more mundane level, we have the ability to decide each and every day how we are going to respond to people and situations. Parts of our lives desperately cry for attention, but we often overlook them until they become a crisis. This alerts us that we must slow down, meditate, contemplate, and seek out support.

My Person Ability staff adheres to an unwritten policy of flexibility and openness. We must be ready to respond and change our plans based on each individual's response to or perception of a situation. There is no single approach in helping any individual. It is important that we are open and able to listen to how we can be of support in any given situation. Sometimes I think our work is simply learning to listen with our heart and not always our head. It's learning how to take a step without being sure where we will land. I have found that when we do this most of the time we find that we land in a safe place. It is equally important to have a continuous desire to learn. We can all learn from one another. By having a strong desire to continue to grow we create opportunities to see things in new ways.

Person Ability's mission is to maximize the potential of an individual or organization. Our logo is a tree formed out of words, with the word "partnership" running down the trunk. We believe that the only way for us to be successful is to develop partnerships with different organizations. The main branches of the tree are formed by the words "community," "culture," "individual," "family," "disabilities," and "organizations." When working with an individual or an organization, one must be aware of each branch while still retaining a holistic view. A tree is symbolic because it represents constant change, with new branches growing and old ones falling off as the tree redefines itself. It is rooted in the community and both gives and takes from its surroundings. Trees are very diverse; each has its own beauty. When we combine the beauty of many trees, however, the power is awe-inspiring and more beautiful than any one tree on its own. Trees provide shelter for others and yet they flourish from the support they receive from their surroundings, through the sun, water, and soil. Because of this, trees have become our metaphor for individuals and organizations.

Each moment in time brings about change while providing both an opportunity for us to become aware of the possibilities for a better personal life and a chance to take a more active part in the larger world around us. Person Ability helps individuals and organizations to open their minds and become attuned to their surroundings. We have the power to create a future that helps us to soar to new heights. We are told how, what, and who to be so often that we forget the innocence we once had as a child, but it is this innocence that can open the window to our mind. What we think about or focus on is ultimately what we become.

Person Ability is made up of a diverse team of individuals who challenge each other's thinking and help those we serve with a variety of perspectives. The majority of our staff are people with disabilities who cross different cultures in society. We are an equal opportunity employer and do not discriminate based on race, age, gender, or sexual preference. Individuals who are currently able-bodied may be just a moment away from acquiring a disability. We feel it is important to try and reflect this in our staffing patterns.

When my husband and I traveled to Peru in 1988, I knew I wanted to climb to the top of Machu Picchu, Incan ruins located nearly 8,000 feet above sea level; navigate through Lima; and maneuver through the jungles of the Amazon. I practiced my walking and ability to climb stairs for six weeks prior to our trip, building up endurance so that I would be able to climb. I knew I would need to make some adaptations to my crutches so that I wouldn't sink into the soft floor of the jungle. The people at the shoe repair shop and I created a five-inch base that widened the bottom of my crutches and worked marvelously. There were some steps along the ruins that were almost as high as my legs are long. I used my crutches as though they were rails to help me reach the top of the spectacular ruins. It was a glorious event. As we climbed through the jungles there were moments when I didn't feel secure. At one point we could only enter our camping huts by walking along a wet tree trunk that had fallen in the jungle. My husband looked worried performing this task, and I certainly didn't feel comfortable doing it on my crutches. Even so, during the middle of the night you could hear my crutches clanking as I wandered down the plank to the outdoor bathroom. I had no alternative, so I overcame my discomfort.

Last summer on a trip to Hong Kong, I presented a speech at an international conference for social workers. I traveled with my husband and a new, hot pink, quickie sports chair* to increase my freedom and maneuverablilty throughout the city. This was the first time I had traveled with the aid of anything other than my crutches. Once again, it opened my eyes to the opportunities, experiences, and situations that nondisabled people take for granted. I feel very blessed and fortunate to have had these wonderful experiences and one of my goals is to be able to continue to travel both nationally and internationally speaking and consulting.

Recent awards with which I have been honored include two from the State Society for Hospital Social Work Directors, one for outstanding leadership and the other for creative programming; membership (along with only forty-eight other individuals throughout the country) into the National Hall of Fame for People with Disabilities; the Advocate of the Year award granted by the Statewide Independent Living Council (SILC); participation in the Statewide Business Leaders Network, the SILC, and the President's Committee for the Employment of People with Disabilities; and an Exemplary award for the National Network for Social Work Managers.

I anticipate my future with the curiosity and excitement of a child. My goals and dreams are to help my children grow, feel good about who they are, help them find their gifts and talents and share them with the world. I plan to continue to travel the world speaking and consulting and learning from others. I also plan to continue to develop my personal and professional rela-

---

*A wheelchair without side rails that has better tires and wheel grips that are easier to grasp than regular wheelchairs.

tionships so as to grow to deeper levels of understanding. I hope that Person Ability will continue to mature and redefine its niche. I would like to someday write a book, finish my doctorate in adult education and continue to find situations where I can facilitate the process of learning. I will continue to help people find their passion and develop the discipline, knowledge, enthusiasm, creativity, and zest necessary to accomplish their goals. I will continue to dedicate my life to helping disenfranchised populations find equality, justice, and the opportunity to live their lives and fulfill their dreams.

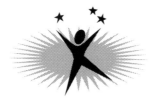

The Littlest Ambassador

Daniella Fortuna

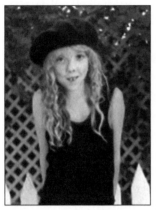

Daniella Fortuna, eleven, suffers from facial disfigurements due to a hemangioma growth. In addition to being a Children's Hospital Los Angeles spokesperson, Daniella was recently selected as a Children's Miracle Network "Champion"—one of fifty-one youngsters picked who have courageously battled deadly or debilitating diseases. She now works as an ambassador for the organization, whose mission is to generate funds and awareness programs to benefit kids and associated children's hospitals in the United States and Canada.

I first realized I had a hemangioma when I was about four years old. A hemangioma is a benign tumor made of spongy connective tissue. They are quite common and vary from person to person, but most are quite small and appear on the upper body. Mine covered almost my entire face. Hemangiomas are the result of a genetic or birth defect that causes tumors to form because there is too much blood for the veins to handle. When I was about two weeks old, red patches (like birthmarks) began to appear on my face. By the time I was one and a half, these patches had become raised and had grown into big, red tumors.

To me the hemangioma was like a red bubble that kept growing on my face. I know my eyesight was affected and I still don't have very good vision in one eye. The side effects of hemangiomas differ greatly, but in my case the tumor was forcing my eye to close and my parents and doctors were afraid I might lose my vision because of it. There was some hemangioma inside my mouth, and so they were also concerned about my breathing. A CAT scan was done to see if there was any hemangioma inside my head, which could have been fatal because it would have interfered with my brain.

My parents talked to me about having a birthmark and surgery and about other children and their possible reaction to me to prepare me for kindergarten. Before that I had heard my parents talk about my condition sometimes but I really didn't realize or understand that there was any problem. Once in a while someone will stare or say something although the birthmark is gone because of all my surgeries. The only thing I have now are some scars, my nose is a little bit different, and I have some dental problems. I probably will have more surgery but my doctor left it up to me to decide when.

My feelings about the hemangioma changed over time because at first, when I was five, I was very scared and didn't like going in the hospital. After my first and second surgeries, though, I got to know the hospital and all the doctors and nurses. I knew what the routine was going to be. I don't like all the needles and surgery and the pain, but it's a little easier to deal with things when you know what to expect. I'm eleven now and I understand that the surgeries are going to make my life a lot better, but I still hate all the needles and the mask they use for the anesthesia.

The most difficult thing about having the hemangioma was the name-calling and the stares. I tried not to let it bother me. There were only a couple of times I can remember when kids made fun of me or called me names. My parents explained that some kids didn't know any better even though it is very rude. My parents said that kids are naturally curious, but we agreed that parents should teach their kids to be understanding about people that are different or handicapped. My mom calls that "compassion." Everyone on this planet has feelings. I think that if someone felt the hurt of being called a name he or she would never do it again. Some people don't realize how lucky they are to have no health problems. I try to not let myself get down about anything. My family is very positive and avoids getting stuck on negative things. Sometimes we try and understand why people act a certain way. We talk about it and then just let it go and go on with our life.

A couple of times I went to the school principal and then talked things out with a classmate who had made a comment, but I really didn't have that many problems at school. I went to the same school from kindergarten to fifth grade and I got to know all the teachers and kids and principal and staff really well. The principal of my school, Dr. Nancy Dean, is really a neat person. She taught me a lot about self-esteem. She always dressed really nicely, wearing beautiful outfits and hats and stuff. She was strict but not mean. She taught us to respect each other. We put on an incredible Christmas show every year. The last year I was there the Christmas show was a copy of the Academy Awards. I got to be the master of ceremonies with one of my best friends, Stan. My mom was always involved at my school. When I met First Lady Hillary Rodham Clinton in February 1996, she gave me a copy of her book, *It Takes a Village.**

---

*Hillary Rodham Clinton, *It Takes a Village and Other Lessons Children Teach Us* (New York: Simon & Schuster, 1996).

My mom read it with me and I now understand what it really means. I feel lucky because I know I've always had a lot of support from my family and friends and from Children's Hospital.

I met my doctor, Dr. John Reinisch, in a very unique way. My parents had been looking for a doctor for me for almost two years. Everyone told them something different—some doctors told them that nothing could be done to help me. My parents were very upset and frustrated. Then one day when I was almost two years old, my dad was playing with me in the front yard of our apartment building. A jaguar pulled up to our front yard and a very beautiful woman named Nancy got out and started talking to my dad. She asked if there were any apartments available in our building. She looked at me and asked my dad if I had a cavernous hemangioma. My dad was shocked because not everybody knew the medical term for what I had. She told my dad that she worked with children who had facial deformities and their families. She said that sitting in the car was a man named Dr. John Reinisch, a plastic reconstructive surgeon who worked on children with facial hemangiomas. They both worked together at Children's Hospital Los Angeles (CHLA). She gave my dad her card. My mom and dad were really glad. (We found out later that they had seen us in the neighborhood and wanted to help us but didn't know how to approach us.) I started seeing Dr. Reinisch right after that, and my mom and dad got involved in Nancy's support group for parents. We still think of this as our own private miracle. Dr. Reinisch is one of the best plastic surgeons in the world and he travels all over the world to help children. He is also my friend and a very nice person.

I try to help other people who are uncomfortable

around those of us with serious illnesses. I want them to see that we can't help the way we are, that there is no reason to be afraid of us, and that we have feelings, just like everybody else. I have a friend, Brandon, who has Down's Syndrome. He was in my fourth grade class. The other kids used to help him a lot. It made him feel good because people cared and it made us feel good that we could help somebody. I have also met a lot of kids at Children's Hospital who had a lot of different illnesses and diseases. I met a girl named Jessica who was my age, at one of the tapings at Children's Hospital.* She had AIDS, and her mother and brother did too. The father didn't have it. They are a very brave family. They went in front of the camera when Jessica was sick and blind to tell their story and help raise money for the hospital. Jessica died earlier this year. It was very sad.

I also met fifty other kids from all over the United States and Canada who were chosen to be Champions across America and participate in the Children's Miracle Network Telethon broadcast from Disneyworld in Orlando, Florida. Every one of them had been through something difficult in their lives. I try to make people understand that someone who is sick or handicapped or something is a person too. We're just kids and want to enjoy life like everybody else.

I got interested in public speaking when I was about six years old and I was asked at one of the telethons to tell the story of what my family and I went through. I

---

*Children's Hospital Los Angeles (CHLA) and the Children's Miracle Network (CMN) produce a lot of videotapes about the different people involved with the hospital. Some tapes feature doctors and their specialities, some are about research, and some feature celebrities, patients, and their families. These are often used to help raise money and promote awareness for the hospital.

really enjoyed telling our story. Taping it was a lot of fun. I met a lot of really nice people, like Steve Edwards, a Los Angeles-based newscaster. Also, when you think about all the people who watch television it makes you feel good about what you are doing. I didn't get too nervous and I like to talk so they kept asking me to do more things for the hospital. My parents said that I was probably helping a lot of people by doing this, and it turns out that I have helped some people. There were two different families from different states with children who had hemangiomas and did not know what to do because they lived in small towns and the doctors there were not familiar with hemangiomas. They saw me on TV, found out about Dr. Reinisch, and came to California to have surgery. I also think that if other kids were watching me on TV and were afraid about surgery and disease, maybe I helped them not to be so afraid. That is what inspires me. The work I've done at Children's Hospital makes me feel good about myself and it is also a lot of fun.

I became involved in Champions across America this year. One child from each state in the United States was chosen to participate. Not all the kids who were chosen were disabled. Some were born with birth defects, but some had overcome or were still fighting diseases like cancer and AIDS, and some had been in accidents. Each child had a different story, and all are champions because they are strong and courageous and are overcoming difficult situations. I was nominated by my hospital. It really is an honor. We went to Washington, D.C., and met the President and the First Lady at the White House. We took a tour of Washington, D.C., and visited all the memorials. We also went to Arlington National Cemetery and some of the kids got to lay a wreath on the tomb of the unknown soldier. Then the organization flew us to Orlando, Florida, to be in the Children's Miracle Network Telethon, which is broadcast nationally each year to raise money for all the children's hospitals across the country. The money is used to buy things like incubators for premature babies like I was, to help build cancer wards, to fund research for diseases like AIDS, and to help buy special needles and equipment because children need smaller medical stuff. The Children's Miracle Network really does a lot, and the people there are really special. Being a part of the telethon is one of the neatest things I ever got to do.

I became a Children's Hospital spokesperson when I was about seven years old. This happened because I like to talk and shared my story with people at fundraising events and they responded to me very well. My duties as spokesperson for Children's Hospital Los Angeles include participating in fundraising events, and through this I've done all kinds of different things. The telethons are the main thing, but I've done a commercial with MasterCard and the American World Cup Soccer team and they gave me a soccer lesson too. I participated in a fashion show with Remax Realty to raise money. I've attended luncheons and dinners with very important people from the hospital. I've been on TV shows and radio shows, attended horse shows, and I was at the finish line at the Los Angeles marathon. I introduced the First Lady at a booksigning/fundraising event in front of 1,500 people. I try to do whatever I can because this is very important to me and it's a lot of fun. I get to meet a lot of really nice people and doing all this also makes me feel good about myself.

I met Hillary Clinton for the first time this year when she was in Los Angeles for a fundraising/booksigning event at the Beverly Hilton hotel in Beverly Hills. Chil-

dren's Hospital sold tickets to hear her speak and atten-
dees received a copy of her book, *It Takes a Village*. Part
of the money raised went to Children's Hospital. The
event took place in a huge ballroom with a big screen for
showing videos and tables set up everywhere. Everyone
was pretty dressed up. It was really crazy for my family
and me because it turns out that I was scheduled to also
make a appearance on the "Leeza" talk show on the same
day. As soon as we were finished with "Leeza," we were
driven to the Beverly Hilton. I was a little bit nervous because the place was so big and there were going to be so
many people there. There were huge lines of people outside the hotel. After I saw my friend Steve Edwards and
he told me we were going to be on stage together I felt
better. What I had to say was a mouthful and I didn't
want to mess up. They showed the video my family and
I had made for Children's Hospital and then I went on
stage with Steve and I talked a little bit about my experience at the hospital. Then I introduced the First Lady.
I was very nervous, but I did it perfectly: "Ladies and
gentlemen, the first lady of the United States of America,
Hillary Rodham Clinton." Mrs. Clinton is really nice.
Some people don't know but she has been raising money
for children's hospitals and children's rights for many
years—long before she became the First Lady. She is also
a lawyer and a really good speaker. She asked me to
come back up to the stage when she finished her speech
and we greeted all those people together. It took hours!
After that we went backstage with the secret service
men and washed our hands together. She met my mom
and dad and invited us to the White House. It turns out
that we were going to see my grandparents in Maryland
in April, so we all got to go to the White House. We got a
private VIP tour. We also went to the secret service

building. I asked if I could see Socks because I love cats, so I got to meet and hold the first cat! We took a lot of pictures and Mrs. Clinton also arranged for the official White House photographer to take pictures. She was very nice to us and I had a great time.

I have met a lot of famous people through the hospital, usually through fundraising events. I'm not too shy so I like to talk to them and take pictures and get their autographs. It's really interesting to meet all these different people who want to help children. They work very hard. I look up to them and want to be like that when I grow up. I met Steve Edwards at the telethons. I met Mayor Richard Riordan at the Los Angeles Marathon, and a lot of the Dodgers baseball team at a celebrity softball tournament. I met Steve Young, Mary Lou Retton, Marie Osmond, John Schneider, Merlin Olson, Coach "K" of the Duke University basketball team, Bo Jackson, and many others at the Champions across America tour. I like all of them and they are all really nice. My most special friendships are with Hillary Rodham Clinton, Steve Edwards, and Steve Young.

I have received a few awards. I have a proclamation from Governor Pete Wilson congratulating me on being a Children's Miracle Network Champion, and of course being the Champion of California is an honor. I have about twenty different awards from school, mostly in language arts and science, which are my favorite subjects. I also have been named student of the month a few times. It feels really great to receive awards. I've been in the newspaper a lot and done a few TV shows, too. Sometimes I'll be out with my mom or dad and people will come up to us and say that they have seen our story on TV. They tell us that our story is really inspiring. Sometimes they say they have been following our story for years and they wish us well. It feels good to know that there are a lot of nice people in the world.

Some of the most memorable people that I have met are kids at Children's Hospital. I don't know if I have helped them, but we shared our experiences and became friends. I think it made us feel like we are not alone, and you get strength from that. I know I've helped some children who heard me talk about not being afraid of the hospital. I met a little girl at the "Leeza" show who had a hemangioma and I talked to her about it. She was really young and scared to be on TV. A few people saw my story on TV and found out about Dr. Reinisch, so I guess I helped them too.

My parents have helped and motivated me in the past because they are very special. They always tell me the truth about everything and they always support me in everything I do. They are always there for me, we talk about everything. My parents are really nice people and they are a lot of fun. We have a very happy life. My mom is very strong and she always tries to be nice even if somebody is rude. Everybody likes my parents. I hope to be like them when I grow up. I really value my family and friends.

I really wouldn't change anything in my life. If I had been born without the hemangioma, maybe my life would have been more "normal," but I wouldn't have gotten to do so many things and meet so many wonderful people. I think having a hemangioma has changed my life by making me aware of some of the things that happen to children, trying to help others and not be selfish and spoiled. I think I have an opportunity to do good things.

In the future I plan to be an actress. I have studied at the Lee Strasburg Institute for over one year, and last summer I studied with a theater group called "Class Act." I love acting I've done about six different performances with Lee Strasburg, including the musical *You're a Good Man, Charlie Brown*. Last summer we did Shakespeare's sonnets and once we did a play on Greek mythology. This session we are going to do *Arabian Nights*. I think I'm pretty creative. I like writing poems. I wrote one for the First Lady and presented it to her when we met in Beverly Hills. I also love dancing and swimming. I want to go to college. I love going on trips and seeing the world. I love the work I do with Children's Hospital and helping others.

If I could communicate one message to people it would be to avoid judging people. Somebody who has something wrong or is different might be the nicest person you ever met. Somebody who may not be perfect and beautiful might make the best friend you ever had.

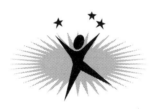

My Ups and Downs:
Living with Down's Syndrome

Ann M. Forts

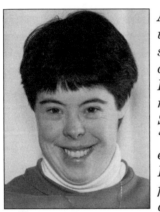

Ann Forts was diagnosed at birth with Down's Syndrome. At the age of seven, she began using a crayon to cross out "Down" on the National Down Syndrome Congress newsletter, replacing it with the word "UP." Shortly afterward she began using her "UP Syndrome" logo on T-shirts, caps, etc., to raise money for the National Down Syndrome Congress. A new fund, called the Annie Forts "UP Syndrome" Fund, was begun early in 1997 to assist people with Down's Syndrome and provide scholarships in special education and related fields. She speaks nationally and has made a career advocating for people with mental disabilities. Forts was presented with the Joseph P. Kennedy Jr. Foundation Award for Self-Empowerment at the United Nations and appointed a member of the President's Committee on Mental Retardation.

I was born thirty years ago on March 10, 1967, in New Jersey. My mother told me I was born on a bright, sunny spring day and my whole family eagerly awaited my arrival. The day after my birth the doctor told my parents that their new baby had Down's Syndrome. Furthermore, he strongly advised that my parents not bring me home but instead immediately place

148

me in an institution. The doctor's recommendation was based on his belief that if I was brought home the family would grow attached to me. He felt it would then be too difficult for them to place me in an institution, even though I would begin having a negative effect on my family. He indicated that I probably would never amount to anything in my community and that I probably would lead a very uneventful life, filled with many disappointments and discouraging situations.

Fortunately for me, my parents did not take that doctor's advice. My family's love for me had grown during the nine months of my mother's pregnancy and it has continued to grow since the day I was born.

I did not know what Down's Syndrome was or that I even had a handicap until I was six or seven years old. I knew that I was different when I started school because I was always sent to schools outside of my town. I was always in classes with other children who had some kind of physical or learning problems. As I got older, I began to realize that there were some things that I could not do very well or at all. It was frustrating and harder for me to learn to do things because at times, the things that I was trying to do either seemed too difficult for me or I just did not understand them.

I guess the worst part of having Down's is that so many people stare at you. In the beginning, it made me feel very uncomfortable. Later, I learned several responses to turn the tables on those who stared at me. For instance, when I see people staring at me, I give them a big smile. It usually surprises them. I walk over to them and shake their hand, introduce myself, and ask them their name. Sometimes I give them my business card and they are surprised when they read that I am a self-advocate and motivational speaker. When they see that I am friendly and courteous, people begin to realize that I am not much different from them.

I am very lucky to have been born into a close and loving family who have lots of fun together and are always happy. The members of my family love life and are always very supportive of me and everything that I try to do. Due to my family's outgoing and positive lifestyle, I naturally began to think and do things in the same confident way.

I was seven or eight years old when I started to think and learn about Down's Syndrome. My family was, and still is, a member of the National Down Syndrome Congress (NDSC). Each month we received the NDSC newsletter, *Down's Syndrome News*. One day I was walking back to the house after I had picked up the mail from our mailbox. I looked through the mail and saw the new issue of *Down's Syndrome News* and thought that using the word "down" seemed a bit negative. Later that day, I was busy drawing and coloring when I again noticed the new issue. I picked up the copy and decided to improve the name by crossing out the word "down" with my crayon and replacing it with the word "UP." Using "down" didn't seem right to me, so for over twenty years, I have been crossing out the "down" and writing "UP" instead.

I don't like to use the term "Down's Syndrome" because, to me, it sounds negative and I have always been an up person. I found out that "down" is used in "Down's Syndrome" because the doctor who discovered the condition many years ago was Dr. John Langdon Down. I really wish his name had been Dr. Up so that today Down's Syndrome could be called "Up Syndrome" instead. If the term were different maybe more people would begin with a better attitude toward those with

Down's Syndrome and they might start to understand who we are and what we are capable of doing.

The most difficult thing that I have had to deal with is that too many people try to prejudge what I can or cannot do just because I have a disability. I want to have the same opportunity to try doing the same things that everyone else does. I might not do some things as well as other people, but I certainly do enjoy myself. I am always willing to try something new, especially when people tell me it is something they think I cannot do. Sometimes, I surprise them and myself as well.

Over the years, the National Down Syndrome Congress (NDSC) has had a very important influence on my family and me. The NDSC is a family-type organization offering all kinds of information, help, and encouragement to people with Down's Syndrome and their families. The annual conventions are great for families and include a separate conference for youths and adults. The conference is very helpful to people with Down's because there are workshops to help us make the most of our lives. We learn about independence, the importance of friends, employment, inclusion, speaking out for ourselves, learning how to express our thoughts and to get other people's attention, and how to set goals and plan for our future.

The NDSC also provides young people with an opportunity to experience serving as a member of the board of directors, which meets twice a year. The board includes three young adults with Down's Syndrome who are elected for three-year terms. Each year a young adult is elected at the Youth & Adult Conference to replace one of the three young adults retiring from the board. By being on the board, we have the chance to offer some of our concerns and complaints. While there is a lot of business discussed at the board meetings that we don't understand, there are many other items that we can speak out about. It definitely is a great experience for us and, I hope, for the other board members.

The NDSC is so helpful in making a better future for people with Down's Syndrome and their families that I decided I wanted to help. I created Ann's "UP Fund" which donates profits from the sales of various items using my "UP Syndrome" design to NDSC. My family helps me set up different items including T-shirts, sweatshirts, tote bags, backpacks, caps, pins, and buttons to sell. Since I started selling "UP Syndrome" items in October 1990, I have donated over $17,000 to the NDSC.

In addition to having served two terms on the NDSC board of directors, I also serve on three other boards. I am in my second one-year term with the New Hampshire American Association on Mental Retardation and a second three-year term on the governor of New Hampshire's advisory council, the New Hampshire Developmental Disabilities Council. I am also serving a three-year term on the President's Committee on Mental Retardation (PCMR) in Washington, D.C.

The PCMR is an advisory committee to President Clinton that has twenty-one members appointed from all over the country. I was one of the first two members with a disability to be chosen. I have heard that there is a rumor around Washington that my appointment is the only one that has not been challenged by Congress.

I am very thankful for the great opportunity to serve on an exciting and interesting committee with dedicated and knowledgeable members and staff. We sponsor forums and discuss and prepare reports and recommendations to President Clinton concerning people with mental retardation. We also publish a quarterly newsletter called *Spotlight*. I am the chair for the PCMR sub-committee on Mission and Public Awareness. The sub-committee is responsible for setting goals regarding issues and needs relating to improving life and opportunities for people with mental retardation as well as for publicizing and distributing the information gained through PCMR's various activities. I feel very fortunate to be able to express my feelings and opinions on behalf of the mentally retarded.

A number of exciting and interesting things have happened to me because of my position on the President's Committee on Mental Retardation. Great things started to happen just before the Christmas holidays when Gary Blumenthal, the PCMR Executive Director, called to tell me to pack my bags and be ready to fly to Washington, D.C. The full committee had an appointment to meet President Clinton at the White House and present two of our advisory reports to him.

The next morning we went through the White House security clearance gate and were escorted by secret service men into the White House Oval Office. The reports were presented and then we each had a chance to speak to President Clinton individually. I introduced myself and he smiled. The President shook my hand and I gave him a press packet, one of my "UP Syndrome" pins, my business card, and one of my "UP" caps for when he goes jogging. I also asked him not to cut the budget for people with disabilities because we really don't have anyone to speak and look out for us. President Clinton said he would do what he could to protect our interests and gave me a big hug.

An hour later, President Clinton gave a speech at the annual luncheon for the Democratic Leadership Council and mentioned me in his speech. Because of that, I was asked to be interviewed by Katie Couric on the NBC-TV "Today" show the next morning. I was then approached to be on the Geraldo Rivera show the next week and then interviewed by both New Hampshire WMUR-TV News and New England Cable News. I was also interviewed by six different newspapers. The best part of all the media attention is that it has enabled me to send my "UP Syndrome" message out to many people.

The excitement didn't stop there. The Moultonboro, New Hampshire, Lions Club decided to hold a huge community celebration on March 1 to honor me and start raising money for my new nonprofit fund, the Annie Forts "UP Syndrome" Fund. The fund provides financial assistance to anyone with Down's Syndrome anywhere in the United States and also provides scholarships to one or more graduating high school seniors who plan to study special education or a disability-related course of study. The celebration on March 1, 1997, was a huge success. Over 500 people attended and after only five weeks, over $48,000 of the initial $50,000 goal was raised. Also, the governor of New Hampshire proclaimed March 1 as Ann M. Forts Day throughout New Hampshire.

With all of the television and newspaper publicity, and having pictures featuring President Clinton, John F. Kennedy Jr., and me at the White House appear in *Life* magazine, my speaking engagement calendar for 1997 is beginning to fill up with twenty-two speeches scheduled so far. Last year I traveled over 26,000 miles and spoke to more than 6,000 people all over the United States.

No matter what kind of group or organization I speak to, my "UP Syndrome" philosophy is always the most important part of my speech. I also include all of the other factors that are necessary for a person with a disability to lead a satisfying, meaningful, and re-spected life in his or her community: independence, mo-tivation, speaking out, community involvement, pride and self-esteem, inclusion, sharing, and volunteering. I speak to many different types of groups and organiza-tions such as parent support organizations, self-advo-cates, teachers, students from elementary to graduate schools, doctors and nurses, local and state social workers, community service organizations, and state, regional, and national conferences.

I enjoy my public speaking career and I feel that I have lots of worthwhile messages to give to many dif-ferent groups of people. I feel certain that my speeches have changed many misconceptions that people have about the Down's Syndrome community's supposed in-ability to lead active, productive, and satisfying lives. Speaking also gives me the opportunity to meet many new people, to make new friends, and to travel all over the United States. I am very thankful to Dartmouth College for getting me started on my speaking career seven years ago. I was invited to speak to a class of al-most one hundred pre-med students about my life growing up with Down's Syndrome. I guess they liked what I had to say, because for the next five years, I was asked to speak to each new class of pre-med students.

My talks to the pre-med students were always on the up side of Down's Syndrome and described my active life filled with many friends, activities, volunteering, and jobs. All my talks included the story about the doctor's advice to place me in an institution immediately after I was born. I close my talks by asking the audience to re-member one question: "Can you imagine how different my life would have been if my parents had taken that doctor's advice?"

It was early in my speaking career that I was asked to give an opening welcome speech to over 1,500 people at a National Down Syndrome Congress annual convention in Denver, Colorado. It was there that I met actor Chris Burke for the first time. He congratulated me on my speech and made me feel very important because he was a big television star on the series "Life Goes On." I was awed by the fact that he was a well-known television actor. I gave him one of my "UP Syndrome" T-shirts.

Our friendship grew each time we met at the NDSC annual conventions. Chris is a very good role model for me and other young people with Down's Syndrome. We admire each other and support each other's efforts to encourage and inspire anyone with Down's or any other disability to do their very best at all times, to speak out for themselves and their friends, and to try to be as independent as possible.

Chris and I have become close friends over the past several years, even though he lives in New York City and I live in New Hampshire. We are able to see each other several times a year when I am in the New York area and when Chris visits his sister who lives in New Hampshire. We also get a chance to meet at different conventions or meetings. I think the reason that our relationship works so well is because we both admire and respect each other for our efforts to show people that with the right attitude and effort, they can have a satisfying and rewarding life.

There are many different things that have helped me overcome the disadvantages of having Down's Syndrome. I am sure that people with other kinds of disabilities will find that the same things that have helped me will also be helpful to them. From my experience, attitude is probably the most important part of being successful and accepted. An up or positive attitude is necessary if you want to improve your confidence or self-esteem. With the right attitude it becomes easier to make friends, and having many friends makes it easier to be included in your community. Inclusion means acceptance and independence. All those things add up to a happy and productive lifestyle. We must learn to speak out for ourselves and make things happen. We cannot afford to waste time by waiting for someone else to make things happen for us. If we wait for someone else then we will miss out on a lot of interesting things. If we don't get enthusiastically involved, we cannot expect inclusion to be a major part of our daily lives.

Over the past few years, I have been surprised to have been honored with several awards. The most famous award that I have received is the 1995 Joseph P. Kennedy Jr. Foundation International Award for Self-Empowerment in the field of mental retardation.* It was awarded at a big, fancy reception at the United Nations in New York City. Previously, there had been six different award categories (scientific research, education, employment, future leadership, community integration, and leadership in public policy). A new category, self-empowerment, was added to the international awards in 1995. I am proud to be the first person honored with the new self-empowerment award. Eunice Kennedy Shriver, sister of Joseph Kennedy Jr. and the late President John F. Kennedy, presented the award to me. I have also been honored with the 1995 Down's Syn-

---

*The Joseph P. Kennedy Jr. Foundation offers funding to encourage new methods of service and support for people with mental retardation and their families and to promote developments to reduce the incidence and prevent the causes of mental retardation.

drome Ambassador of Good Will Award from the Association for Children with Down Syndrome; the National
Down Syndrome Congress Special President's Award
and two Honorary Service Awards; the 1997 Dr. Allen
Crocker Annual Award presented by the Massachusetts
Down Syndrome Congress; the 1997 Spirit of the ARC
Annual Award from the Association of Retarded Citizens
(ARC) of Union County, New Jersey; and the Lions International Community Service Award. It is a very satisfying to receive an award. More important, I feel satisfaction in being involved and getting enjoyment out of
actually doing the things that people and organizations
want to reward you for. It is like getting paid for a job
that you really enjoy.

Sometimes parents of people with a disability come
up to me after I have given a speech and tell me how
much I have helped them. Many are people who had
heard me speak before, talked to me previously, or read
about the things that I have been doing. I try to impress
upon everyone the importance of love, attitude, friends,
getting involved, volunteering, making things happen,
independence, pride, trying new experiences, doing your
best, speaking out, and setting goals.

When I think about my life and all of the great
things that I have experienced, I definitely would not
want to change anything because I am having too much
fun the way my life is going. In fact, I think that I have
a much more interesting and satisfying life than most of
the people I meet who don't have a disability.

I value the love of my family and the many friends
who share their time and support with me. I know that
without the constant love and support from my family
and friends, I would not be enjoying my life the way I
am today.

Although I am leading a very active and interesting life, I have some very important goals that I would like to reach. They include writing my autobiography; continuing my speaking career throughout the United States and expanding it internationally; helping to make inclusion, with respect and without reservations, of those with disabilities in schools and communities a reality; and to reach my ultimate goal of $1,000,000 in donations for the Annie Forts "UP Syndrome" Fund.

People ask me what is the most important message that I can pass on to them. My answer is to learn how to develop and maintain an up attitude most of the time. A positive attitude is the foundation for all the good and necessary things needed for an interesting, satisfying, and productive life filled with love, friends, support, inclusion, and respect.

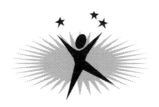

A Champion for Children

Kathryn Petros

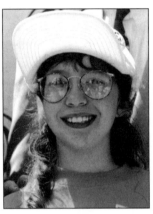

Kathryn Petros was diagnosed with acute lymphocytic leukemia when she was seven years old. She was chosen as the Children's Miracle Network Champions across America representative for Alaska for her many projects that help other children. To describe her cancer treatment, Kathryn wrote the short story "Chemo is . . ." which is distributed at children's hospitals in Los Angeles and Alaska. She has also appeared on the Children's Miracle Network Telethon and the Petros family volunteers for the Make-A-Wish and American Cancer Society foundations. As a Champions across America representative, she has visited the White House, met President Clinton, and participated in the Children's Miracle Network broadcast from Walt Disney World, Florida.

I am now eleven years old and I live in Anchorage, Alaska. I am a sixth grade student at Chugach Optional Elementary School. I am involved with many charities and belong to the Girl Scouts. In May 1993, when I was seven years old, I was diagnosed with acute lymphocytic leukemia (ALL). My parents first noticed my symptoms in the spring of that year when I kept getting strep throat. As soon as I finished my medication, the strep throat would come back again. My immune system was not strong enough to fight infections. I developed a staph infection* in my finger and was back at the doctor's office. On Saturday, May 21, I had planned to perform in a dance recital with my tap class. I woke up with my eye swollen shut and a high temperature. My mother took me to the doctor's office once again. My parents thought I had contracted pink eye, but the condition was soon correctly diagnosed as dermatitis, an infection caused by an insect bite near my eye. My mom described all of my symptoms to the physician's assistant, who decided to test my blood. The nurse pricked my finger. A few minutes later she came back and said she had to do it again because the first test did not "work." After the second test they told my mother that I was very anemic and had very few red blood cells, the cells which transport oxygen throughout the body. I was going to have to go to the hospital and have complete blood work done on the following Monday.

After we went home, I took some Tylenol and took a nap. When I woke up I felt better and decided to dance in my recital that night, but afterward, I was very tired. The next morning, I slept until after 11:00 A.M. and woke with a temperature of 103.3°F. My dad called the doctor's office and they told him to meet the doctor at the hospital as soon as possible. My dad still thought my problem was pink eye. The emergency room doctor checked me out and said pink eye was not the problem. Then a nurse came and took a blood sample from a vein in my arm. By this time, one of my own doctors had arrived. I remember her talking to my mom and dad, saying that I was very sick. They were going to have to

---

*"Staph" is short for staphylococcus, a type of bacteria that is very common in skin infections.

do other tests to find out why I had a fever and why my blood count was so low. My mom called my grandmother and had her talk to the doctor because my uncle has Black Diamond Hypo-Plastic Anemia, a hereditary blood disorder they thought I might also have. After the doctor got a thorough family medical history, she called in a hematologist,* who decided I was going to have to have what is called a bone marrow biopsy. A bone marrow biopsy is where a thick needle is pushed into the center of a bone, usually a hip bone, and they draw out some bone marrow. The nurse in pediatrics gave me a shot so I would not feel any pain. I was sick, tired, and scared. My dad stayed with me to hold my hand. I cried a lot. I also had to have a nurse come put an IV in my arm. A few hours later, my doctor came back with the hematologist. They told my parents I had irregular white blood cells, but they didn't think I had ALL. My mom was relieved to hear that even though at the time she didn't know what ALL was. She was just happy that whatever it was, I didn't have it.

I was put on heavy doses of antibiotics and told that I would probably have to stay in the hospital for a while.

The doctor came to see me the next morning and told my parents that he believed I suffered from abnormal white blood cells and therefore was unable to fight off infections. We live in Alaska, and there were no pediatric hematologists in the state who could evaluate my blood work and bone marrow samples. My doctor told me to get comfortable and be prepared to stay in the hospital about a month, or until I was strong enough to stay healthy; my lab work was going to have to be sent to Seattle, Washington, to be evaluated.

*A hematologist is a doctor who specializes in disorders of the blood and blood-forming organs.

I spent the morning getting to know my nurses and the hospital child life therapist, a person who helps kids deal the stress and anxiety associated with hospitals and illnesses. Nurse Emily gave me a stuffed animal, a cat I named Emily, that I still have today. Carol, the child life therapist, gave me a doll and a journal to keep during my hospital stay. Later that day we received the bad news. My doctor had looked at my bone marrow again with the hospital pathologist and they thought they saw very early markers of leukemia. I was flown to Children's Hospital Los Angeles right away.

I didn't understand everything that was happening, I just knew I was leaving. My mom told my doctor in Anchorage that she wanted me to go to Children's Hospital Los Angeles because we had family there and because my uncle had been treated there for his blood disorder when he was young. Because I was so sick and would require medication during the long flight, a nurse had to fly with my mother and me to California. The next day, my dad took my little sister, Kristina, to my cousin's house in California. My aunt and my grandmother would take turns staying with her while my parents would stay with me at the hospital. I rode in an ambulance from the airport to Children's Hospital. When we got there it was very late at night. My new nurse gave me an IV and took more blood. That night I met Jason. He was fourteen years old and had bone cancer. He was a funny guy and interesting to talk to. Later, Jason would become the first person to make me smile when I wasn't feeling very well.

The next day, I met many new doctors and nurses and received many pokes. I definitely was not happy with needles sticking me all the time. Right away I was scheduled for tests, a spinal tap, and another bone marrow biopsy. Luckily, they would put me to sleep for these tests. The next evening the doctors gave my family the diagnosis. My Uncle Paul stayed with me and played video games while my parents went off with the doctors to have what they called their "Biology 101 lesson."

The bad news was that I did have cancer, acute lymphocytic leukemia. The good news was that it had been caught very early. Doctors put you in one of three categories when you are diagnosed with leukemia: poor, moderate, or good prognosis. I was labeled "good prognosis" with an 85 percent chance of being cured. My parents were overwhelmed, but at the same time determined to help make me well again. One thing I have always appreciated and admired about my parents is that from the very beginning they promised to be honest and up front with me about my illness.

On Friday, my sixth day in the hospital, my parents came to see me with the doctor; Elva, the child life therapist; and Dr. Hudson, the hospital psychiatrist. They explained that I had a blood disease called leukemia. My blood wasn't making enough good white blood cells and the "blasts," immature or mutated white blood cells, were overpowering the good white blood cells, crowding them out. Blasts take over the bone marrow and prevent it from making enough blood cells, including white and red blood cells and platelets, causing anemia, bleeding, and infections. That is why I kept on getting sick. I was also told that I was probably going to get sicker before I got better. I was going to have to take all kinds of medicines that would have unpleasant side effects. I needed the medicine to kill the bad cancer cells in my blood. I felt sick and I couldn't eat anything. I was tired of seeing the nurses come with the needles to take blood or give me medicine. I would cry, scream, and tell them to go away. I would say I had to go to the bathroom and try to stay in there until they went away, but they never would go. I was angry and upset with everyone and everything.

Before I got sick, I had hair down past the middle of my back. The doctors had explained that the job of some of my medicines was to kill cells. Some would kill not only cancer cells, but hair cells too. My long, beautiful hair was going to fall out. I forgot about the cancer. I couldn't go to school or let my friends see me bald. I could have cancer, but having my hair fall out was not acceptable to me.

Soon, the doctors, nurses, and therapists helped me learn things to make everything bearable. My doctor tried a new cream called Emla, which the nurses would put on my veins before taking a blood test or inserting an IV. The Emla numbed my skin and I didn't feel the needles poke me.

Dr. Hudson and Elva explained that when my hair fell out, I would know that the medicine was working and killing the bad cells to make my cancer go away. My bald head was my badge of courage. Dr. Hudson taught me tricks to relax during treatments and how to breathe slowly during spinal taps. He helped me learn to swallow pills. Elva let me perform tests on rag dolls in the play-room. I gave dolls spinal taps, bone marrow biopsies, and IV's. This helped relieve my tension and anxiety.

My parents bought me hats, hats, and more hats, so that when my hair began falling out I wouldn't feel self conscious. They were also given many ideas on how to handle my hair loss. They were told to shave it all off to get it over with, or to cut it very short. My Grandma Petros and Aunt Sue suggested putting my hair in a ponytail and cutting my hair off just above the ponytail, then they could glue my ponytail to a hat, and I could still "have" my hair. I decided that I wanted to keep my hair the way it was as long as I could. When my hair began to fall out, I began wearing my pretty hats.

After two weeks in the hospital, I was allowed to go home, which meant my Grandma "J's" house in the San Fernando Valley. We were going to have to stay in California for three months, or until I was in remission. My mom and Kristina would stay with me, but my dad was going to have to go back to work in Alaska. He worked for a company that had flight benefits and was able to come see me on weekends. He would come to some of my clinic visits, and at night he would read to me to help me understand my cancer.

Finally, I had finished my "induction therapy" and was allowed to go back home to Alaska. The first phase of chemotherapy was over, and it felt so good to be in my own home, sleep in my own bed, but mostly, to see my friends. I was going to have to go back to California for the "reintensive" phase of chemotherapy, a second stage of treatment during which I would receive stronger doses of the chemotherapy drugs, so I wanted to spend a lot of time with my friends while I was back at home.

When I left Los Angeles I had the protocol or "road map" I was to follow for my treatment while I was in Alaska. Life became an endless round of doctor visits, blood work, and hospital days for chemotherapy. My mom also had to go back to work while we were back home. My parents worked for the same company in the same department. They started having problems at work because their schedules conflicted and their boss said staying home with me was a daycare problem. My dad ended up switching to another division of the company, one more willing to schedule his work around my mom's hours. They worked opposite shifts so one of them could be home with me all the time. I felt responsible for everything. Not long afterward I decided I was tired of being sick. I cried and cried and told my parents that I wished I was dead so their problems would go away. They knew we had to make big changes at once. First, I got a great counselor to talk to who would listen to my problems. Mom and Dad stopped arguing about work and we decided we would think happy thoughts.

Because of my illness and some of the medicines I was taking, my immune system was suppressed, which means that my body couldn't fight off illnesses as well as other people's could. In an effort to to keep me from catching colds, I was not allowed to go back to school when it started in September. Every week I had cell counts done to see how my blood was functioning. The results determined how much I was allowed to do. Even though there were many things I was restricted from doing, my parents told me to concentrate on what I could do. They told me I had cancer, not "don'tcer." We needed to focus on fun things in life. I could still take ballet. I could still see my friends if they weren't sick. My school offered French classes after school. Because it would be a small group, I could take French classes with my friend Molly. I could still go fishing or hiking with my dad.

If my counts were high enough I could visit my class at school. On the days I would visit school, the kids and some parents would always ask me questions. Thankfully, my parents always kept me informed on my condition and my treatments so I could usually answer their questions. My friends did not fully understand chemotherapy. Some of the parents thought chemotherapy was radiation treatments. I decided to write a short story titled "Chemo is . . ." about chemotherapy for a writing assignment. My mom wrote down my words and I drew the pictures. I described my different types of medication and procedures. Someone once asked me about spinal taps, and if they hurt. I told them because of the Emla cream there was no pain, just some pressure, "kind of like an elephant stepping on your back." My mother made extra copies of my story and gave them to the doctors, psychiatrists, and child life therapists at both Children's Hospital in Los Angeles and at Providence Medical Center at home. I have been told that they have been able to share my story with other new patients. Kids need to know they can be involved in their treatments and help make choices about how they do things.

Soon it was time to go back to California for the reintensive phase of therapy treatments that were not available at home. The medicine was much stronger this time and I felt very sick and weak. I received many cards and letters from the kids in my school, friends and family, and even from people I didn't know. Receiving the mail cheered me up. It helped to go to the hospital in a happy mood. Once I got a card that came with special stickers in it. I "wore" the stickers on my back when I went to the clinic for my next spinal tap. One sticker said, "use no hypos here" and the other said "THIS END UP." Humor and love went a long way to ease the burden of my illness. I started looking forward to seeing my nurses, my doctors, and the child life therapist.

After I finished with the reintensive phase of treatment I went on "maintenance," a chemotherapy regimen that is followed for a period of two to three years in a three-month cycle. The maintenance cycle for me included IV medication, pills, antibiotics, steroids, and spinal taps. Soon after I started maintenance, my hair slowly started to grow back. I wore my hats everywhere. People always knew who I was because of my hats. I was grateful that my friends never treated me any differently because I had cancer. I never felt like someone's science project. My parents told me that because I had self confidence, people didn't notice the illness. I was a regular kid who just happened to wear cool hats and had cancer.

I had a great "visiting" teacher who came to my house to teach me. We tried to follow the same lessons my classmates were studying. My mother was always giving me extra assignments or buying me workbooks. My sister, Kristina, who was two and a half, would have coloring books and we would all sit at the dining room table to do our schoolwork. My mom said that just because I wasn't in school it wasn't an excuse to sit around and be lazy. We were going to take advantage of the time I had at home. There were days off for chemo visits, or when I was too weak or sick to work. We took things one day at a time.

The Christmas before I had cancer, my mother and I had been walking through the mall. We stopped to listen to a harpist play holiday music. I loved the music and the harpist reminded me of an angel. I decided to ask Santa Claus for a harp. I didn't get a harp that year. My dad said Santa really didn't have room for something that big in his sleigh. The next Christmas came and I still wanted a harp. My parents told me again that I probably wouldn't get one because Santa didn't think that seven-year-old girls really wanted to play the harp. Sure enough, Christmas morning came and there was no harp under the Christmas tree. After all the presents were opened, my dad handed me a note from "Santa." He wrote that many people were proud of me and that they had asked him to send me a special present. After several minutes, I found a strange package hidden behind one of my sister's presents. It was a harp! (Later I found out that friends of my parents had all gotten together and bought the harp for me.) In January 1994 I started taking lessons on my folk "lap" harp, which has nineteen strings. My harp teacher is the same lady I had met in the mall the year before. I have been playing the harp for three years and I now rent a harp that is much larger and has thirty-four strings. Skookums (my teacher) has always given me encouragement and support. Learning to play the harp has taught me love, patience, and beauty. Sometimes I would bring my lap harp (which I can play sitting down, with it in my lap, or sitting on a small stool, with the harp on the floor) with me on my school visits. I enjoy playing for my friends and family.

Once, when I was at the hospital in Alaska for chemotherapy, I saw my harp teacher playing in the lobby for people. The next Christmas (1995) I decided to give a harp performance to thank the nurses for taking such good care of me, and for the families of sick children in the hospital. I had spent the previous Halloween and Easter in the hospital and it was very depressing, and I wanted to do something to make the holiday more cheerful. I learned some Christmas carols and helped my mom bake some cookies and other treats. Mom taught me how to make some decorations that I gave the nurses. I had a great time treating the nurses and playing my harp. People came from all over the hospital to hear me play. I was featured in the local evening news. I continue to play at Christmas every year.

I had been on the receiving end of so much kindness, I wanted to give some back to others. In June 1994, the people at Providence Medical Center asked me to tell my story during the Children's Miracle Network Telethon. I had been interviewed by the news before and enjoyed it. My family and I had such a positive experience and appreciated the quality of care I received at the hospital that we agreed. The local NBC station sent a reporter to our house. I played my harp. My story ran throughout the local portion of the telethon. I also got to answer phones to take pledges during the telethon and sell Children's Miracle Network balloons and T-shirts in the lobby of the hospital. It was a fantastic day for the whole family. I learned that sometimes it is just as important to give of yourself and your time as it is to donate money. My family volunteered to help at the next telethon. The local news came to the hospital to videotape my chemotherapy appointment. I had IV medication and a spinal tap. They filmed me with Carol, my child life therapist. We showed how I would give chemo to her special dolls before I had mine. Children's Miracle Network supports the child life therapy program and helps provide quality care to all children, regardless of their ability to pay. Funds also help provide medical equipment for hospitals so they can help kids with special needs.

In September 1995, I went back to Children's Hospital Los Angeles for my end of treatment exam. Again, I was put to sleep for a spinal tap, a bone marrow biopsy, and other blood tests. The results showed that I had achieved complete remission! I was off all chemotherapy medications. I would have to take antibiotics for another year to help my body fight infections until my immune system was back to normal. We didn't have any parties to celebrate, though, because unfortunately, my spinal fluid "leaked" during the exam and I was very sick for the next week. I returned to the hospital four times to receive IV fluids so I would not get dehydrated. It wasn't quite the end of treatment we had expected, but it helped to remind everyone how fragile life is. After all, I have to remain healthy for a total of five years after the end of my treatment without a relapse before being considered cancer-free.

I was able to go back to school full time when I came back home to Alaska. I didn't have to take any medicine to make me feel sick. My parents could just be my parents, and not doctors or teachers. My sister, Kristina, missed having me around at home all the time. She was used to having all day for us to spend together. She had helped take care of me when I didn't feel good and held my hand when I got poked. She looked out for me.

When I was undergoing treatment I was lucky enough to have a wish granted by the Seattle chapter of the Make-a-Wish Foundation. I wanted to see dolphins. I think they are one of the world's most beautiful creatures. Make-a-Wish sent my family to Hawaii, where we went deep sea fishing and parasailing. On my special day, Kristina and I had an exciting time playing with the dolphins and staff at Dolphin Quest at the Hilton Waikoloa Resort. I got to pet and feed the dolphins. We played ball and I got them to do tricks for me. My family was relaxed and happy. It was a dream come true. A picture of me kissing one of the dolphins is posted on the Seattle Make-a-Wish website. My family became very involved in our local Make-a-Wish chapter. My mom is a volunteer and helps grant wishes for other children. My dad helps to meet families that come to Alaska have their wishes to granted. We all help at fundraising events, selling T-shirts, handing out brochures, or speaking about our experience with the organization.

We also support the American Cancer Society's "24-

hour Strides against Cancer" marathon (now called "Relay for Life"). Runners collect pledges and run laps in groups over a twenty-four-hour period. I have participated every year since 1994. The first time my family participated we ran on my doctor's team. My doctor was impressed with my running ability, despite my illness. Last year, my children's cancer support group, the Soaring Eagles, had their own team. I went door-to-door collecting pledges for the American Cancer Society.

The Leukemia Society of America participates in marathons all over the United States to help raise funds for research and patient aid. They match leukemia patients with runners, enabling them to meet and become pen pals. It provides a great incentive to the runners and helps to put a "face" on the disease. I have met many wonderful people who have run in my honor. Every summer in Anchorage we have a Mayor's Midnight Sun Marathon. It is one of the many marathons in which the Leukemia Society and their Team-in-Training runners participate. In the past, our support group has helped out by manning an aid station, passing out water and wet sponges. It was fun and exciting to cheer the runners as they passed. This year (1997), I am hoping to participate by either running or walking in the half-marathon. I will be matched with runners from Alaska and Seattle. I know I'll definitely be there to cheer them on. My father has recently joined the Team-in-Training program and has begun training to run his first marathon in my honor in December 1997 in Honolulu, Hawaii.

In 1996 I received an honor from Providence Medical Center at Anchorage, Alaska, and the Children's Miracle Network (CMN). The theme of that year's CMN telethon was to celebrate children who had overcome medical hurdles—they called us "Champions." I was selected to represent Alaska as their champion, along with one child from every state and the provinces in Canada. Our job was to represent the over 7 million children helped at Children's Miracle Network-affiliated hospitals. As a CMN champion, I appeared at locations selling the Children's Miracle Network balloons, or at businesses having their CMN kickoff campaigns.

All the CMN champions and their families traveled to Washington, D.C., and Orlando, Florida, to participate in the Children's Miracle Network "Champions across America" broadcast from Walt Disney World. In Washington, we toured the city and visited Arlington National Cemetery. A few of the CMN Champs were chosen to lay a wreath at the tomb of the unknown soldier. We had lunch on Capitol Hill where the CMN Champion broadcast was officially kicked off by Steve Young of the San Francisco 49ers. I also met Bo Jackson, Mary Lou Retton, and other sports stars. All the families had lunch there and some of us had an opportunity to meet our state representatives. We met so many wonderful families, strong kids and parents who had gone through tough experiences and come out champions after their illness or accident. Later that afternoon we were all guests at the White House. All the champions were gathered together in a receiving room, with our families off to the sides. First we were greeted by Hillary Rodham Clinton, who gave a short speech and greeted us. She shook everyone's hand and talked with each of us. We weren't allowed to have our cameras in the White House, but both CMN and the White House photographer took pictures for us. It had been a long, hot day in D.C. and Kristina fell asleep by the time we were inside the White House. My mom tried to wake her up when Mrs. Clinton came into the receiving room, but she would not wake up. She had wanted to see Socks, the president's cat, but my parents told her that she would probably not be able to meet him. One of the Miracle Champs asked Mrs. Clinton if we could see Socks, and soon Socks was in the room. We all got to see and pet the first cat. He was very soft and gentle. My mom tried to wake Kristina up again, and for Socks, she woke up. She slid right out of my mother's arms and under the ropes to join the champions gathered around Socks. Finally President Clinton came out to greet us. He shook our hands, spoke with everyone and took lots of pictures. It was quite an honor meeting President and Mrs. Clinton. It was a thrilling day.

That night we flew to Orlando for the CMN Champion broadcast. We had fun going around Disney World in the morning. I been selected along with seven other champions to be in a parade at MGM Studios with a CMN celebrity. My parents dropped me off at the start of the parade route and went to wait for me at the end. I rode on the back of a 1950s Chevy convertible with the CMN champ from New York, Minnie Mouse, and CMN co-founder Marie Osmond! I had a lot of fun riding around and waving at everyone. At the end of the parade, there was a ceremony where we got to put our handprints and sign our name in cement with the celebrities. This will be installed in MGM's Walk of Fame. One day my family and friends will be able to walk along and see my name and handprints in cement at the MGM Studios. Also, all of the Children's Miracle Network champions were presented with medals. The front is engraved with "Convention of Champions 1996" and the back reads, "Thanks to CMN champs, the kids always win" with

Together
Everyone
Achieves
More. (TEAM)

Participating in the CMN telethon was a unique experience. It was a fantastic opportunity, and I met many wonderful people. I write to all my new friends at CMN. Last year when I visited California, I got together with CMN Champ Daniella Fortuna, whose story is told earlier in this book. We went to the movies and shopping at the mall. It was fun. I can't wait to visit her again on my next trip to California. As a result of being a CMN champion, I have been interviewed on the news and in the newspaper in the "Alaska Achievers" column. I was also featured on the local segment of "Radio Ahhs," a nationally broadcast children's theme-based radio program, usually found on AM stations.

I have a neighbor named North who is a few years younger than me. We both had the same type of leukemia. North finished his treatments soon after I finished mine but unfortunately, he relapsed and needed a bone marrow transplant. He and his family had to move to Seattle until a bone marrow donor could be found. I went back on the news and "Radio Ahhs" to help get some community and emotional support for North and his family. Kids from all over wrote to North and his sister, sending them letters and pictures. My mom and I visited the school he attends. We talked to teachers and students about North. We discussed and answered questions about having cancer. North received his transplant and I hope he returns home this summer.

This year at school our class has had several community service projects. We supported a homeless shelter for the holidays and we ran a school store to raise money for the Children's Miracle Network (CMN). We also had an ice cream sale and used that money to rent a dunk tank at the CMN carnival in our hospital's parking lot the day of the annual telethon. I gathered my friends together to answer phones on the telethon that night. We stayed past midnight and afterward had a sleepover at my house. It was fun! My class hopes to help out at this year's champions broadcast from our local hospital.

I have been so blessed to have met so many wonderful caring and helping people. I can't help but want to give something back myself.

Even if I could change one thing about my life, I wouldn't change anything. I have learned so much and having had cancer is a big part of who I am today. What I value most is having my life and the support from my family. I know their love and encouragement saw me through some of the tougher times when I was very sick. Having had cancer only changed my outlook on life a little bit. I just have to remember to keep myself healthy, and not do anything crazy like smoking, drinking, or doing drugs.

I have been in complete remission for two years. My health is very good. I enjoy riding my bike, reading, writing, hiking, skiing, swimming, and fishing with my dad. I enjoy having parties and hanging out with my friends. I still play the harp and want to record some children's music for the new Children's Hospital at Providence Medical Center. I think harp music is very relaxing and soothing. My plans for the future include becoming an actress or a model. I also want to continue to help sick children. My message to people would be to stay healthy, and stop the violence.

PEACE, LOVE, AND HAPPINESS.

You may make contributions to Children's Miracle Network at:

Children's Miracle Network, 4525 S. 2300 East, Bldg. 202, Salt Lake City, Utah 84117, or by calling (801) 278–8900, or, you can contact your local CMN-affiliated Hospital.

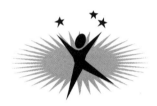

The Cycle of Success

Pam Fernandes

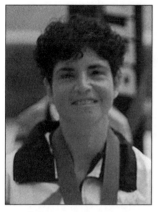

Pam Fernandes is one of seven children and was born and raised in Stratford, Connecticut. She has had Type I diabetes since the age of four, which has led to the complications of blindness and kidney transplantation. Pam's spirit and determination have helped her endure more than thirty operations and come out a winner. She is one of the world's finest tandem cyclists, having won a silver medal in the 1994 World Championships and, most recently, a bronze medal at the 1996 Atlanta Paralympic Games. Additionally, Pam volunteers her time as an advocate for education and research in diabetes. She has become a prominent speaker and, in addition to her many other awards, she was nominated for the O'Leary Award, the highest honor given to an athlete with a disability.

Physically challenged? Who, me?

I am legally blind and have struggled with diabetes since I was four years old. I have exercise-induced asthma, GYN pre-cancer (a growth of abnormal cells which, if left untreated, could lead to cancer), and

I wish to acknowledge the assistance of John Caher, state editor for the Albany, New York, *Times Union* and co-author with James P. Caher, Esq., of *Debt Free: Your Guide to Personal Bankruptcy without Shame* (New York: Henry Holt & Co., 1996).

I've survived some thirty operations, although I did "die" twice. Osteoporosis is thinning my bones. My gall-bladder is long gone and I've got a stranger's kidney. Somewhere along the line I had a stroke, or so the CAT scan says. I guess I'm every health insurance company's worst nightmare. But physically challenged? I hate the phrase. We're all challenged in one way or many, and my challenges haven't prevented me from becoming a world-class athlete.

That's right. World . . . class . . . athlete.

Since my first season racing tandem bicycles, I've been on a roll, literally and figuratively, capped by a medal-winning performance at the 1996 Paralympic Games in Atlanta, Georgia. In addition, I'm a four-time national champion and silver medalist at the world championships. Along the way, I've collected numerous honors, including being named Female Athlete of the Year by the United States Association of Blind Athletes and Athlete of the Year by the U.S. Olympic Committee in 1994 and receiving the New England Women's Leadership Award presented by the Daniel Marr Boys and Girls Club of Dorchester, Massachusetts. I was honored with the 1994 Massachusetts Governor's Award for Physical Fitness and Sports and was one of fourteen athletes nominated for the 1995 O'Leary Award, which recognizes the achievements of outstanding disabled athletes in America. I've been featured in *Sports Illustrated,* the *Boston Globe,* the *Albany Times Union,* and dozens of other magazines and newspapers, appeared on nationally televised shows, and have become a fairly popular motivational lecturer.

I was particularly honored to speak at the Champions in Life Program organized by the White House and the U.S. Olympic Committee in May 1996. Although the event wasn't actually at the White House, it did culminate with a memorable incident when a stranger approached and shook my hand. "Who are you?" I asked him. He responded, "Bill Clinton." Oops! As you might expect, I was a tad embarrassed, but the president was very pleasant and understanding. After all, I couldn't see him.

All of this attention is somewhat unnerving, since I don't think of myself as someone special. What scares me about doing interviews is the possibility that the article will be written from the angle of the poor, pitiful, disabled person struggling heroically to maintain a life that's not worth living. That's not me and it's not my attitude. My overall attitude is positive, upbeat, and uplifting—and I think my speeches reflect that. There's nothing as rewarding as helping another person achieve his or her potential, whatever it may be and whatever his or her limitations. And we all have limitations.

What I have found is that people, both disabled and able, seem to use me as a barometer, a motivator. They think I have accomplished something they could never do. But I want people to stop looking at me as somehow gifted or talented or strong. I'm not any of those things. I'm just someone who plays the cards she was dealt, makes the most of what she has, and tries not to dwell on what she doesn't have.

You just don't know your strength until you are challenged, and it's possible that if you're not challenged you never become a complete person. If someone had told me when I was fifteen that I was going to go blind, lose my kidneys, have thirty operations, and have GYN precancer, I probably would have jumped off a bridge. I wouldn't have thought I could handle it. But I can. I once heard somebody say that God's gift to you is your life, and your gift to him is what you do with it. I think that's right and I'm determined to be the best that I can be. I'm also confident that my mom's admonition is correct: God only gives you the crosses you can bear.

I was born in Stratford, Connecticut, in 1961. At the age of four, I was diagnosed with Type One, insulin-dependent, diabetes. I only remember knowing I had to take a shot every day and that I wasn't supposed to eat sugar. I suppose I knew most of my life that I could go blind. I used to sneak into my parents' room and read about diabetes in the encyclopedia. By the time I was eighteen, I still had perfect vision. Nothing hurt. There was no indication to me that anything was going wrong. So I figured I was pretty safe.

Then my world came crashing down. I was just about to start school at Wheelock College in Boston when my ophthalmologist told me I had some small hemorrhages in my eyes. "Nothing to be concerned about," he assured me, "but you should see a specialist when you get to Boston." Three weeks later, he sat me down and said, "You are going blind." In diabetes, the high glucose (sugar) concentrations in the blood cause aneurysms (bubbles or blood-filled blisters) of the blood vessels in the retina of the eye. Even with laser surgery to remove the aneurysms, the retina is eventually unable to get enough nutrition and it ceases functioning. In my case, scar tissue also formed and the retina ultimately became detached, leading to vision loss.

I remember crying a lot when I heard. It's pretty tough to take news like that, especially at the age of twenty-one. Within about a year or so, by 1982, I was legally blind, unable to perform tasks I had once taken for granted, simple things like walking to the mailbox or making a pot of coffee. I began my transition into the world of blindness, learning to read and write Braille, finding my way around with a cane. While learning to cope without sight, I discovered that my kidneys were failing. Aneurysms were developing there also, resulting in the loss of function.

At that point, I was beginning to feel like the biblical character Job, the good man whom God repeatedly tested. When I was a kid, I thought, it stinks to be a diabetic, but it'd really stink to be blind. Then I went blind and I thought, this really stinks, but I can live with it. At least I'm not on dialysis. Then I had renal failure. What next? What did I do to deserve this?

Exactly one week before my twenty-second birthday I began dialysis. Three times a week I needed a three-hour, often painful dialysis treatment. For five years, I either made regular treks to the hospital for the treatment or did it at home. I found the leash far too short and finally decided I just wouldn't live that way. The limitations dialysis placed on my body were far too great, and in my mind, the only way out was a transplant. I decided to take the risk.*

Before a donor was found, I had to have my gallbladder removed. A day and a half after surgery, I stopped breathing. I remember waking up, gasping for air, not knowing where I was, but knowing I was at the center of something very, very bad. That was the first time I died and came back, an experience I would encounter again medically on one occasion and athletically on many occasions.

---

*Anyone who receives an organ transplant must take immunosuppressant drugs so that his or her body will not reject the "foreign" organ. The suppressed immune system is then less able to fight off infections, increasing the possibility of complications from other sources, such as bacteria or viruses.

On October 21, 1987, I successfully received a kidney transplant. Within a couple of weeks, I was asking the doctors if I could start exercising. They told me to wait six weeks, but I started stretching and doing sit-ups at home. I wanted to make my body do what I wanted it to do. For too long, doctors and circumstances had limited my life, and I'd had enough. So, I joined Fitcorp, a corporate fitness center in downtown Boston, and met the owner, Gary Klencheski, an impressive and inspirational person who got me started on a sensible exercise routine. Gary and his staff were confident in my abilities and their confidence boosted my self-esteem. They expected a lot from me, as much as from any other member. They understood I needed an outlet, a goal, something that made all those hours in the gym worthwhile.

I come from an athletic family. My sister Patty, one of my six siblings, is player-coach for a world championship softball team, and my brother, Butch, is a black belt in Tae Kwon Do. All my siblings were active in varsity sports. I had been a pretty good high school basketball player. I had always enjoyed physical activity, so when a thoughtful cyclist called the foundation where I was working and offered to pilot a tandem bicycle, I jumped at the chance.

Cycling gives me an incredible feeling of freedom. When I am on the bike, there are no barriers, no boundaries that, if you let them, can become all-encompassing. When I walk on the street, I'm always listening for things, always on my guard, always on the defensive. But on the bike, I feel as though I am breaking through all those barriers, focusing on something—anything, everything—other than my disability. I'm so grateful to the rider who got me started. I remember the euphoric feelings of freedom I had on that first ride, and how I wanted to go faster and faster, not to run away from my disability, but to defeat it in head-to-head competition.

Shortly after that first ride, I called the head coach for the U.S. Association of Blind Athletes, Peter Paulding, and he encouraged me to attend a training camp in Colorado Springs in 1993. It was there that I met Mike Rosenberg, a national-caliber cyclist and exercise physiologist from Eugene, Oregon, who had the enthusiasm, unbridled energy, and demeanor of the Tasmanian Devil. We hit it off immediately and I asked Mike to pilot for me at the 1993 nationals in St. Louis, a race open to anyone, not just a special event for the disabled. To his surprise, and mine, we won.

I suppose our racing styles are similar, although I didn't know that the first time we raced. We both like a high cadence, or quick, pedal speed. We both climb hills well. I suppose we have established a relationship that goes beyond racing. It is understanding. It is trust. It is confidence in each other's ability. I trust him and I suppose he has to trust that I won't give up on him. Mike seems to know my capabilities. He pushes me as far as I can go and, at times, a little beyond. He will sometimes temper me if he thinks I am going too hard. But he never gives up on me, is never condescending, and he fully expects me, as his racing partner, to pull my weight. I think he would say I do just that.

As I mentioned, we won the nationals in St. Louis, the first race we entered, and we did it despite the fact that we live and train 3,000 miles apart. We have proven to be an extremely strong duet, routinely winning races for blind athletes as well as open competitions. One of our most memorable races was the sixty-four-kilometer road race at the 1994 World Championships in Ghent, Belgium. When we were warming up,

I remember Mike saying, "I feel good, *really* good today," which gave me a boost in confidence. We were spinning around, getting the bugs out and before I knew it, we were at the starting line. The start was very quick and for a while there was no communication, just pedaling. Suddenly, Mike called for "more power in the turns." I didn't realize at the time what was happening, but I eventually learned that we were trailing an Australian pair. They were braking before the turns, so every time they turned, they would slow down. We had to slow down too and were getting dropped from the pack. Before Mike realized what was happening, there was a pretty good gap between us and the lead pack of about seven bikes. That's the nature of bicycle racing, a sport that combines the sheer determination of a marathoner with the tactics of a chess master.

"We're attacking in town," Mike said. So we bided our time. Mike monitored the other teams and I motored in the rear, and finally the push was on. I got myself ready for what I knew would be a long, hard effort. As we sped through the town, chasing down the lead pack to bridge the gap that had opened, I heard the cheering crowds.

"We're on!" Mike said. We caught them.

The cagey Spanish team that had been in the lead figured out our strategy and attacked as soon as we caught up. Since we were tired from the chase, we got dropped again. But Mike and I geared up for another surge and, once again, caught the Spaniards and the other leaders. They promptly dropped us again and we started working with the French and German teams. With about four miles to go in the race, we caught the leaders once again. "Are you ready? Do you have the killer instinct?" Mike demanded. He reminded me that it was the World Championship and wanted me to have the hunger to win.

"Yes!" I grunted.

Racing demands stamina, skill, and determination. On a tandem, it also demands a unique level of communication between the pilot and the stoker. We communicate in little more than grunts. It's Mike's job to keep me apprised of what is going on in the race. When he says "power," I know it's time to push. When he says "we're on," I know we're where we ought to be. When he says "uh, oh," I know that he's about to make some technical adjustment, but I never worry about crashing.

In Belgium, we were going all out when we got squeezed into the curb, a potentially disastrous occurrence at 30 mph, but Mike pulled us out of trouble in time for the final sprint and we gave it everything we had. Finally, I felt Mike let up, reach behind him, and grab my hand. "Second!" he said. The Spaniards had edged us by half the length of a wheel, but we were medalists in world class competition.

Mike and I continued to be successful. We won scores of races, often beating the so-called able-bodied riders and proving that we were a formidable pair, winning four national championships even though we continued to train on opposite coasts. In 1995, we set our sights on making the 1996 Paralympic team.

The Paralympic Games are the second largest sporting event in the world, trailing only the Olympics. Just after the Olympic games close, the Paralympics begin at the same venue. They are overseen by the Olympic Committee and run by the International Paralympic Committee, and have been held since 1960. The competition is intense, but we figured we had a good shot to make the American cycling team.

We started our quest with a first-place finish in the Paralympic one-kilometer time trials in Colorado Springs, followed by a victory in the three-kilometer trial and two second-place finishes in the road race and the match sprints. We qualified for four events and set an unofficial world record in the one-kilometer race.*

The games in Atlanta in August 1996 were an athlete's dream come true: raw athletics, the true Olympic spirit, and an opening ceremony that you didn't have to see, only feel, to appreciate. It was exciting as paraplegic mountain climber Mark Wellman scaled a ninety-eight-foot tower, carrying the Paralympic torch between his knees and doing the equivalent of several hundred pull-ups as he literally rose to the challenge and lit the flame. It was moving as actor Christopher Reeve welcomed all of us, 3,500 athletes—yes, athletes, not pitiful creatures of misfortune—proudly representing 120 nations. As athletes, we communicated in our own way, and language differences proved to be no barrier at all. I would find myself laughing, then suddenly crying, then laughing again. It was as much an emotional and spiritual experience as an athletic one, and perhaps the truest reflection of the Olympic spirit.

What was supposed to be our best race—the one-kilometer event, where we had earlier set an unofficial world record—proved to be nerve-wracking, to say the very least. We were out warming up and when we got back to the velodrome (the cycling venue), somebody yelled out, "You guys are next." Apparently, the events

---

*To qualify as an official record, the event must be electronically timed and monitored by an official from the Union Cycliste Internationale (UCI), an international cycling governing body. Such an arrangement must be scheduled prior to the event and we had not done so.

were a bit ahead of schedule and we went into a panic. We had the wrong bike—a road bike, not a track bike— and the wrong helmets. With the help of our athletic trainer, I sprinted down to the race staging area in my cleats and Mike rushed to get the track bike. We frantically got prepared to go, and then they called a delay, announcing a fifteen-minute warm-up. Still, when we finally did get a chance to compete, our adrenaline levels were in the stratosphere and we raced to a bronze medal performance. Before the games were over, we had placed in the top five in every event—the only male/female team to achieve such a feat.

The terrific year was capped off by my marriage to a wonderful man, a cyclist named Paul Miller. We train together. We commute to work together. We race together. He's a great man and a terrific friend. One of the things I think is so wonderful about Paul is that he doesn't think of me as a person with a disability, just a person. He's got a particularly good ability to walk in another person's shoes, which makes him uniquely sensitive and understanding. When we first met I could tell, even without seeing him, that I had his undivided attention. I knew his eyes and his mind weren't wandering away. Just as he doesn't view me as an invalid demanding constant care, I certainly don't view him as a bandage for my wounds.

During my cycling career, I have increasingly viewed bike racing as a metaphor for life. I have learned a lot about how to handle different aspects of my life and my marriage through the discipline of cycling. In my cycling, I have to set goals and I have to work very hard. I have to evaluate my progress. I have to believe in myself. I have to accept losses when they come, but use them to help me in the next situation. I have to be a team player, summoning strength when it is needed and displaying support when it is called for. I think those are all things applicable to life in general, not just bicycle racing. When I speak to kids, I always tell them that I never go to the starting line expecting anything but a victory because if I anticipate a loss—if my expectations of myself are not what they should be—I will certainly be a loser, no matter where I happen to finish in the pack. Their response is incredibly heart-warming and encouraging.

After one presentation, I received a letter from an eleven-year-old boy who had been in the audience. I hadn't met him personally, but his letter indicated that I had certainly reached him personally. "You do not let your disability stop you from doing anything, especially riding a bike," he wrote. "You just try your hardest and you accomplish it. That proves that even though you have a disability you will not let it interfere with what you love to do." Well, that's true enough. But he melted my heart with the next sentences: "I have a disability, too," he confided, "but it is different than yours. My disability is a learning disability and that makes it harder for me to learn. I want you to know that you taught me if I work hard for what I want, I can do what I love and my disability does not have to stop me."

Because I didn't let diabetes or blindness stop me from cycling, this kid was motivated to be the best he can be, to climb whatever mountain is in his way. What he doesn't know is how much he helped me. In my moments of weakness, when things aren't going well and I start to feel as though I'm on a never-ending road, I think of him, and I know that if he can make it, so can I, and if I can make it, so can he.

My illness, juvenile diabetes, requires constant monitoring and daily insulin shots. Some 16 million Americans suffer from diabetes now, and that number grows by about 650,000 a year. Diabetes is the leading cause of adult blindness. Not only does diabetes affect a lot of people, it also costs a lot of money—according to the National Institute of Diabetes, Digestive, and Kidney Disease, about $92 billion annually, which includes the cost for disability payments, time lost from work, premature deaths, and the direct medical costs for care. So there is an economic, as well as humane, incentive to wipe this disease off the face of the earth. I've traveled to Washington five times to testify on behalf of medical research for diabetes. I hope that that, more than my cycling, will be my lasting legacy.

I volunteer for lots of causes and am committed to doing what I can to eradicate diabetes. I'd love to see diabetes go the way of polio and I am hopeful that a cure is at hand. Although I hold a full-time job and spend a lot of time training and taking care of my husband and son, I make time for important volunteer efforts. For instance, I volunteer at the Joslin Diabetes Center and have chaired the Equal Access Subcommittee for the Governor's Committee on Physical Fitness in Sports. Education and research are the keys. Despite seventy-five years of research, we have not yet found a cure for diabetes. Many promising studies are underway and researchers are optimistic, but diabetes research must compete for both time and funding with many other diseases. Education, however, has shown diabetics that they can survive the disease if they are willing to self-manage it. Intensive control of blood glucose levels, proper diet, and exercise result in lowered risks of diabetes-related complications.

For me, diabetes is much harder to deal with than

blindness. Once you get used to using a cane, a talking computer, or accepting the fact that you can't see, it is always the same. I have learned I don't need vision to be happy. If I am blind and racing, well, so what? I'm on a tandem. My pilot can see. I think people perceive blindness as much worse than it is and, I'm sure, they don't think diabetes is as bad as it is. Diabetes, however, is a progressive disease that changes every day, sometimes every hour. It is continual work monitoring my blood sugar level and I never get a break from it. Every day and every race presents a whole new set of variables. Being blind is no bed of roses, but at least it doesn't change every day, and it doesn't get any worse.

We need to ensure that funding is available to achieve the goal of a world without diabetes. I may not be around to see that world. My brother, Mark, died of complications from diabetes when he was only thirty-three years old. A lot of people are going to go blind or die before this battle is over, but I am going to do whatever I can to make sure that someday another little girl won't be running to her encyclopedia to learn about her perplexing disease. People tell me I am passionate and driven, and they're right. A lot can happen. Diabetes has taken my sight, my kidneys, and my brother, and it could cost me my life. But if the disease thinks it can steal my dreams and my spirit, it's met its match.

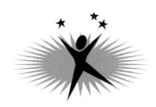

Crossing the Bridge
from Autism to Freedom

Donna Williams

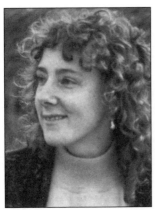

Donna Williams wrote the New York Times *bestseller* Nobody Nowhere, *an autobiography about her life with autism. It follows her journey from childhood as a severely withdrawn and bewildered autistic toddler to a university-educated, successful writer. She speaks worldwide to help people understand autism and recently finished writing several other books.*

I was born in 1963, back in the days when children "like me" were thought deaf, disturbed, backward, bad, or crazy, and at various times in my life I was considered each of these things.

Not much was known about autism back in the 1960s, and many health care professionals in that era had never even heard of it. For many people born autistic in the 1960s and earlier, the only label which stuck was a vague, one-size-fits-all "disturbed." It wasn't until the 1980s, when I was twenty-five years old, that I was finally diagnosed as "autistic." Even by the 1980s, though, professionals didn't have a very clear view of what "autistic" meant. Some called it a communication disorder. Some called it a cognitive disability, and others called it a behavioral disorder. Some saw it as part of an inherited personality disorder and still others called it a developmental disability. No matter how they defined it, they all associated it with certain stereotypes and assumptions.

Autism was something I couldn't see. It used to stop me from finding and using my own words when I wanted to. It made me use all the words and silly things I didn't want to say. Autism used to make me feel everything at once without knowing what I was feeling, or it cut me off from my thoughts so that I believed I thought nothing and wasn't interested in anything. Autism also made my mind almost explode with the need to reach out and say what I thought or show what I was interested in. But often nothing came out, or what came out was contrary to what I'd felt or intended.

Autism used to cut me off from my own body so I felt nothing, and it sometimes made me so aware of what I felt that it was painful to be conscious. Autism sometimes made me feel that I had no self at all. I felt so overwhelmed by the presence of other people that I couldn't find myself. It also made me so totally aware of myself that it was like the whole world around me became irrelevant and disappeared. Autism was my seesaw. When it was up or down I couldn't see a whole life. When it was passing through in the middle I got to see a glimpse of the life I would have if I were not autistic.

I spent my first twenty-five years playing both sides of two battles: a battle to join the world and a battle to keep it out. Sometimes, information overload and sensory-perceptual problems made the world appear to be the cause of my overwhelming feelings of being chaotically out of control, too rawly exposed, in a state of inconsistency where it was hard to find cohesion. When I felt like this, I sided with the anxiety and battled to close the world out. When I felt suffocated by the way my condition robbed me of expressive freedom, contorting my expression or cutting me off from it, I sided with the rest of the world and battled against my world of autism. This endless conflict affected my development in the most pervasive and intimate way, right down to shaping my very identity.

My environment also played a major part. Some people demanded that I function without regard to my true developmental level. Some struggled to join me on a personal and emotional level on whatever terms it took, regardless of whether this meant aiming below my functioning level. Some were ashamed of the reflection my behavior had upon them. Others found me "different," "special," or "entertaining," all of which shaped who I was, usually not in a constructive way. The most important thing I learned was that even though I often sided with it and identified with it, *autism was not me.* It just controlled the expression of who I was. In fact, because of the autism, until a few years ago, I didn't realize that people commonly refer to themselves as "I." I'd always thought of myself in the third person, as "Donna," or simply "she."

Close your eyes and imagine there is only sound. There is the sound of gravel under your feet, leaves crunching, a comb running through hair, and the tinkle of chandelier crystals. There is another constant sound, with an unpredictable rise and fall in pitch and no rhythm. All of these sounds fall upon your ears with equal value. None of them has meaning. Some are pleasant, some are painful, some cause emotional excitement, but none makes any real sense. This was how I heard the world.

Open your eyes and block your ears. Look at the pattern and order of the things you see, the dancing of light and shadow, the teasing variations in the color of things around you and unpredictable dancing faces full of invasive, meaningless expectation pulling themselves into a myriad of seemingly random expressions, flying hands, unpredictable body movements. And all of these sights have equal value. None of them has meaning. This was how I saw the world.

Imagine that meaning does get processed, but unconsciously. You do not know you are intelligent, knowledgeable, or even sane. Reaching for the meaning of things is like reaching into darkness. The darkness is scary so you don't reach in, because if you reach you will find the sense of something terrifying in its foreignness and so much the worse for its inescapable proximity. You will find emotional reaction and an experience of self. But you won't be able to interpret these either, so you will assume that this is what terror feels like. Finding those feelings and that sense of self must be death and must therefore be avoided at all costs.

Imagine you discover suddenly that music flows from your fingers without any learning and painting flows from your brush without instruction, and that words appear on a page caused by keys on a typewriter at which you happen to sit. You are terrified by your words as they appear on the page when you have not even thought them as they were typed. This is the terror of communication, which can be overwhelmingly exposing for someone with autism. The more direct and the more personal communication is, the more threatening it is.

I spent my life communicating obliquely, via songs, commercials, pieces of stored conversations and accents. As a child I parroted whatever the voices of those around me said, hoping that that would make the voices stop. Later, I started speaking indirectly to people by addressing my shoes and hoping that "the walls really did have ears" but wouldn't force me to notice. I remember suddenly discovering when I was thirteen that people did not always literally mean what they said and did. I didn't know the word "superficial" so I used the closest word I had for "false," which was "plastic." I was very frightened and disturbed by this realization but couldn't tell anyone or discuss it. I would walk past whoever I wanted to tell and look at the wall or my feet. "All the people are plastic," I kept saying as I slapped my face to show I felt hurt and frightened. Mostly, people around me didn't understand and thought I was crazy and just talking to myself. If they had forced me to see what I was doing they would have cut me off from my words and I wouldn't have been able to hold the thought or put it into words at all. Only without awareness could I escape the prison of autism into freedom.

I learned to talk using characters or personae. I would step into these characters as though putting on a well established puppet show. Slowly, I found I could speak about things. I could discover my mind as long as I never acknowledged it was me who was doing it. I was able to write a book because I did not think about it. My mind was allowed to attribute the expression to a machine speaking to the paper. It wasn't me. It was the typewriter keys. After my book was spewed out onto paper, in a four-week exorcism, I finally had a picture of a whole self who had lived a whole life.

The rules for communicating with people with autism are not the same rules for everybody else. Non-autistic people need to learn new rules and new methods. Parents and professionals should not assume that if an autistic person does not speak or show reading comprehension, then he or she cannot communicate. Even when these forms of communication are not possible, other forms are sometimes used that nonautistic people may not see or hear. Communication can mean setting up a pattern of rhythm, an arrangement of beads, or notes played on an instrument. Such patterns can develop into a dialogue, either by adding to each other's things or by creating parallel patterns nearby.

The sharing of smells or sounds or textures or colors back and forth in a pattern of give and take can also be dialogue. It enables us to express an awareness of and share in each other's particular sensory-perceptual experiences. It is about reassurance, understanding and confirmation of "me too." It says "we're okay." "Normal" is to be in the company of someone like yourself.

Autistic people are speaking to you. We have always been speaking to you. We have spoken in the language of behavior, in the language of thought, in the language of smell, color, sound, rhythm, pattern, and texture. We have spoken in the language of order, symmetry, and symbolism. We have spoken in the language of mirroring, of autistic metaphor and visual word-pictures. We have spoken through objects, through music, through movement, through art, and through computers. And we have spoken in silence, through an intent gaze or lack of it.

Nonautistic people have much to learn from us. If they spoke nonautistic language it would be easier to know why people with autism have so much to learn from them. We need them to dialogue in a language that needs no translation. That language is understanding. That language is hope. That language is acceptance and support. People with autism need light in the darkness and sound in the silence, bridges in place of walls. We need encouragement to cross those bridges one step at a time from our own worlds to a shared world in which it is safe not merely to appear but to . . . simply Be.

It has taken me almost three decades to finally know the simplest of things—to experience myself and another person essential to the concept of "social." It took me forever to learn to be with someone without losing the sense of one or the other; to listen to someone without struggling to decipher the meaning of clearly heard sounds or trying to look like I was interested when the meaning had dropped out; to know what it was to see a face with the nose within the meaningful context of the eyes and mouth and cheeks without losing the meaning of each fragment as I moved to the next; to know what it was to feel an emotion without perceiving it as an attack purely by virtue of it dragging me back to a body and consciousness I'd rejected in the chaos of its inconsistent messages back in early infancy; to have consistent thought and feeling simultaneously and not have to do all my thinking through objects or on paper; to have been able to speak and hear myself with meaning simultaneously; to know what it was to acknowledge a relationship between myself and another person if only through a spontaneously felt "thank you," or saying their name without being attacked by involuntary impulses to avoid, divert, or retaliate. Those would have been luxuries. And yet, I am lucky. I entered autism at one end and, with a lot of strategies and space to untangle my bucket full of jumbled jigsaw puzzle pieces, and an overhaul of my biochemistry, came out the other. Many haven't.

I spent my first few years totally meaning-deaf and meaning-blind, unable to tell where physical or emotional sensations were coming from or what they were. I spent most of my life tortured by involuntary aversion, diversion, and retaliation responses caused by my own acute exposure anxiety, often unable to acknowledge even to myself that I existed, had a thought, or wanted something. I was unable to acknowledge these things before others without being compelled to disown the thought, the feeling, the half-initiated action or expression and thereby being judged by those involuntary responses. I spent the first years and many years to follow caught up in the grip of emotional flooding, where unprocessed, undifferentiated emotion would tumble down upon me seemingly from out of the blue with no capacity to understand, resolve, or ask for help. I spent my first years being physically attacked by my own body whenever my mind pushed my will further than it could stand, being jolted into awareness of my own existence.

I can't say those years were pure hell because they were also pure heaven. That's the sanctuary of the prison. That's life as a fairground where a lack of meaning can be a world of beauty in a time before the system of interpretation, before the time of mind.

Later, when meaning began to trickle in, it was just enough to be mighty confusing. It was enough to feel tortured by the incapacity to hold on to meaning, to be constantly thrown out again and again by a world of meaning you cannot hold—meaning within yourself and of yourself and meaning relating to sound and sight and sensation from the world around you. This loss of meaning which comes with shutdown due to overload is a punishment, a brutal, repeated abandonment, which you did nothing to deserve but get anyway.

Then came compliance and suppressed terror of discovery that someone would see beyond the apparent "success" of well-trained robotics, to see that true, connected underlying development was fragmented and partial; a one-year-old, a three-year-old, a five-year-old, all within a teenage and then adult body. This was change from the outside, the sort of grace from which one sometimes falls in what gets called "regression," which is really the exposure of one's true level of development when the crap gets dropped by the wayside.

For eight years, from the age of twenty-four, I received treatment for severe digestive problems affecting my ability to regulate blood oxygen, blood glucose, and vitamin-mineral levels which had led to violent reactions to some foods and chemicals. In my case, I believe treatment began to change things from the inside. I'd spent my whole life making emotions and body-connectedness redundant, fighting it and all who would trigger my on-line experience of this perceptual system, often like a matter of life or death, like a matter of war. Now, all of a sudden, this system was looking in whether I liked it or not. I couldn't keep it out. The jolt of conscious awareness which comes with feelings as part of the package was mercilessly on my door step, ready or not, here I come. I was twenty-five and this was the death knell to what I'd known as "my world." At twenty-five, the steel walls of my autistic world were melting.

I needed to get everything out of me and put it all down on paper so I could hold it all together without letting exposure anxiety force me to avoid the awareness that emotional thought would bring. I felt that if I could get it all out of me then I could take it all back in and own it. I could outrun the invisible robber within me which compelled me to tune out anything, such as awareness, that would jolt my feelings. I also felt that if only I could hand it all to a therapist of some sort then that person could tell me why I was like this and tell me how to fix it.

Words had never worked. As soon as other people gave me their track, I lost my track and went on theirs. Maybe, in writing, my track would hold itself in place and they'd see me, instead of me reflecting their idea of me.

In a compulsive and obsessional four-week do-or-die purge, I let out of me the automatic typing of my first book, *Nobody Nowhere.** I was unable to think a single sentence. I didn't plan the structure of the book. I didn't seek the memories. I just sat down and let it out like a big, typographical vomit.

Every night I'd come home from the clerical job I was currently holding with such a grip of dread, like I was facing death, and it was death, it was the death of the reality I'd known, a private and evasive reality, even slippery to my own grip.

I read my life back off the pages as they became typed and tears kept falling without sound. In silence, I screamed my life out onto paper from my strangulated mind. After four weeks, when it was done, I read it all as a whole book and knew for the first time who I'd been and what I'd lived. I became free to think, free to remember. Now, if I was to be free before others, I had to allow myself in book form to be experienced by at least one other person in the world. If one person had experienced it, such a person could conceivably pass on that knowing to anyone anywhere. If I could do that, exposure anxiety could never trap me again. There'd be no possibility to hide, either from myself or from others. That one person read it and asked that it be sent to a publisher. I accepted that as the way to be free of what had kept me imprisoned all my life; the "exposure anx-

---

*Donna Williams, *Nobody Nowhere: The Extraordinary Autobiography of an Autistic* (New York: Times Books, 1992).

iety" arose as a result of information overload which left my body connectedness off line to the point where I developed an aversion to all experience of it. This was a major part of what others called my "autism."

Through the eventual publication of *Nobody Nowhere* the nonautistic world went on a journey from a position about as close as it gets—a private book written from me to me, a last dash for freedom as the final speck of hope seemed almost lost. That book freed me, a person terrified of exposure and the consciousness and emotion it triggers, to live with myself with awareness and, further, to live this before others. I set it free into the hands of the world in the hope that it would free me from my crippling terror of self-exposure, not before others, but before myself. In the years that followed, I learned that it also led to an explosion in the diagnosis of people with autism. A condition once defined by narrow stereotypes about low-functioning people perceived as having a dim prognosis is gradually giving way to seeing these people within a much broader continuum, one that holds much hope.

By chance, at the age of twenty-five, like so many others born in the ignorance of the 1950s and 1960s, I was correctly diagnosed. Not deaf, not mad, not disturbed. I was autistic.

In the years that followed, I wrote my second book, *Somebody Somewhere** and tackled my remaining sensory-perceptual problems and became the master of the compulsive state that arose from a life of feeling plunged into endless inconsistency and robbed of control.

In *Somebody Somewhere* I mapped my first steps, ex-

*Donna Williams, *Somebody Somewhere: Breaking Free from the World of Autism* (New York: Times Books, 1994).

posed and freed before a world I'd been too reactive to be-friend, and introduced the world to a whole range of people across the autistic spectrum as well as the trans-lation between autistic and nonautistic reality.

In writing about others like me, I wrote of Ian, a man with whom I developed a "specialship." I also developed a system of relating I call "Simply Being." Through my "specialship," and later, marriage, I became friends with emotions and learned to recognize the real self from its many hiding places. This formed the third of my sequels, *Like Color to the Blind*,* a book which finally took me to that fine line between autistic and nonautistic realities.

Somewhere in there, I also allowed the world to touch the writing most sacred to me from late childhood into adulthood—my poetry and songs, published in the book *Not Just Anything*.†

In the seven years since writing my first book, I have had so many letters asking so many things, I decided to answer not just those who wrote but all those who didn't. I wrote the self-help book *Autism: An Inside-Out Approach*.‡ I wrote it so people won't have to keep suf-fering from ignorance and hopelessness, so families of people with autism and people with autism themselves can have something they've been missing—empower-ment. I wrote the book the professionals should have, a book about the mechanics of autism, problems of con-nection, problems of tolerance, and problems of control.

---

*Donna Williams, *Like Color to the Blind* (New York: Times Books, 1996).

†Donna Williams, *Not Just Anything* (Arlington, Tex.: Future Horizons, 1995).

‡Donna Williams, *Autism—An Inside-Out Approach: An Innov-ative Look at the Mechanics of "Autism" and Its Developmental Cousins* (London; Bristol, Penn.: J. Kingsley Publishers, 1996).

I wrote of autism in all its forms and faces, all its phases and degrees, its adaptations and its facades, but I wrote it so everyday people can read it.

All people can find aspects of autism within themselves. That's because autism is like looking at "normality" under the magnifying glass—when the volume is turned up to an extreme high, inherited traits which would otherwise be harmless are seen in an exaggerated, often dysfunctional form. Even now, in this age of apparent enlightenment, if, as sometimes happens, a child seems to outgrow the developmental effects of autism in childhood, many parents decide never to tell such children they are/were autistic. They dread, despite the improvement, a sudden rediagnosis such as Asperger Syndrome (a high-functioning developmental "cousin" to autism). But this results in the myth that autism is "incurable," and helps keep these people dependent, not speaking, not making friends or having relationships, or whatever. It's about time this myth is retired and people get the tools to build bridges from hopelessness to hope.

By exploring the connections among the various findings to do with biochemistry, nutritional approaches, and autism and having access to all this information because of the success of my books, I found the links between the information available and an approach that existed for the treatment of information processing problems.

The insufficient supply of nutrients to the brain such as vitamins, minerals, blood glucose, and blood oxygen can lead to information overload and the sensory-perceptual adaptation I call "systems mono," a state in which sensory systems are used in a nonintegrated, one-channel-at-a-time way. By having one system on and one system off I'd get meaning through my eyes but become meaning-deaf as a result. Or I'd tune in to meaning through my ears and lose all connection to my body. The experience of total loss of control and the redundancy of the uncomfortable system of body connectedness was so inconsistent that it became invasive when it came on line in the form of feelings, which resulted in the instinctual aversion to conscious awareness of my own expression, which I call "exposure anxiety." When pushed beyond the realms of tolerance, it resulted in the involuntary aversion, diversion, and retaliation responses which are seen as "autism."

Mega-vitamins, special allergy diets, and enzyme supplements became partial answers to these developmental catastrophes in my life, helping me to process information more fully and be less "mono" and more "multitrack." I could begin to use my systems in more of an integrated way and get to know body connectedness. But beyond all this, I came across an existing treatment for the underlying causes of vitamin-mineral and enzyme deficiencies and severe food and chemical allergies, a treatment which had already been used extensively with adults who had postviral fatigue but was generally not used with people with autism, which had long been considered a neurological problem.

Information processing doesn't always have to be about a messed up car or brain. It could also be the result of a messed up fuel system. Some people aren't brain damaged, they are brain affected. It can happen that if the fuel system gets messed up before the age of three, when sensory-perceptual systems are fixedly integrated, one of the adaptations to information overload caused by a messed up fuel system is the splitting off, or disintegration, of these sensory-perceptual systems and its developmental results, something otherwise known by nonautistic translation as "autism."

Several months into the treatment for vitamin-mineral deficiencies, I experienced, at the age of thirty-two, consistent sensory-perceptual integration for the first time in my life. I could process visual and auditory information simultaneously without accumulative meaning-deafness or meaning-blindness stepping in. I could process my emotional responses and was able to differentiate my physical sensations without losing body-connectedness because of overload. I could hold thoughts all strung together in my head. I could simultaneously express myself and monitor what was coming out. I was no longer meaning-deaf or meaning-blind to expression which came from myself, no longer having to double check that I'd made sense or stayed on track. My level of exposure anxiety came down dramatically. I no longer had the overload-induced adrenalin rushes that resulted in sensory heightening. I had consistency and I no longer felt robbed of control. I was now interacting meaningfully with others rather than battling with the strait-jacketed boundaries of my own inescapable condition.

I started up a consultancy to train professionals, assist parents in home-based programs, and help people with autism cope better with their condition. With specialists who could actually treat the biochemistry side of things, I believed I was in a position to help others with autism break through their prison walls. My new venture hasn't been operational for long now, so it's hard to tell how it will go. I've heard some pretty encouraging news so far—a child who has finally begun to speak, another whose daily screaming has stopped, and another who is finally sleeping soundly. One person with autism has stopped attacking herself, and one has stopped attacking others.

I've come a long way in my own war with autism. I earned a college degree and learned how to entertain people with my performances of their "normality." Then I brought my true developmental level out of the ashes and up to being in sync with the functioning level I'd achieved but hadn't been able to experience. This brought a peace I had never known before and the will to live a life I was able to feel and identify as mine.

If I could change one thing in my life, I'd bring back for a day all those who weren't able to see me with this freedom I have now—my paternal grandparents and my father, who died just six weeks before I discovered consistent multitrack processing. I have managed to get a hold of all the others who mattered to me and to be with them as a whole, freed self, to say sorry where I felt it and to say I'd loved them where I'd been unable to show it before.

What I value most in life is clarity, peace, freedom, and enough consistency within which to feel safe enough to let growth happen. For that I credit belief in the light within myself—the life force in all people, creatures, and things which we can each follow or fight or ignore. Mine has led me home and it is my best friend, greatest confidant and source of direction and security, which no change can shake off. Some might call this God.

Autism has deeply affected my values and outlook on life. It made me prioritize. I have no time for the cheap trash of negative game playing or ego-mongering, for people offloading on me emotional or psychological baggage that isn't mine to carry, or for status trips or power games. Having spent so much time just fighting to get past interacting with my condition so I could live my life, autism gave me the greatest appreciation of the preciousness of time. I seize life with a driving force that is sometimes bigger than I am. Autism taught me to do things while I can because nothing stays on line. Its constraints motivated me to be an expert escape artist. It gave me a talent for planning tactical maneuvers to combat developmental mazes. Autism made me perceptive about structure and systems, and compelled me to be objective in order to distance the jolt of awareness and emotion. The mechanics of autism is my version of mathematics, and I am a genius with the intricate system I know intimately with almost absolute objectivity. Autism taught me about war and about the value of love and the many ways of making it palatable. Autism taught me which people were worth the effort and which were not. At the end of the day when the struggle to make it through another twenty-four hours is temporarily over, and you look at who and what is left, you see who the beautiful people are; you determine who needed a "cause," something to fight for for the sole purpose of saying they are fighting, and who really put their own needs and assumptions in their back pocket and put their energies into real understanding and helping of others.

In *Nobody Nowhere*, Lawrie Bartak, the psychologist who diagnosed me, wrote that this book was a story of a life just beginning. It's been hard growing up in the limelight and sometimes it hurts a lot. It's hard to go from three to seven to eleven to sixteen when you are twenty-five, twenty-eight, and thirty-two and you're moving in a world which assumes so much by your adult appearance. But it's also helped to feel the support of the whole world as the family that I shared it all with. One of the loveliest letters I got was from a reading group in Canada who read my first book together and upon finishing it threw a party and baked a cake saying "Congratulations

Donna" on it. These things made me feel safe and gave me assurance that people were trying to understand and valued me and knew how hard I was trying.

I'm learning now to take time out for a personal life. I have a cat called Monty that loves me and he's my good friend. I hope his spirit doesn't leave his body but I guess it will one day. I'll have more personal friends by then.

I spend time getting used to freedom. I'm sculpting, which I wanted to do for twenty years but couldn't because it dared so much expression that the exposure anxiety it caused meant I was always diverted from doing it. Now I've gotten free of that. I did a life-size bronze sculpture bigger than me. She's called "My World, The World," and she's naked before the world staring at her own little world held up in her hand and not realizing that with the other hand behind her she is pushing out the influence of the world around her. She is a statement of the experience of autism, of its hypnotic nature and of its cost. She is my way of placing in time where I was and where I am now and what it took to get me here.

If I have a message for people, it would be something relevant not just to autism but to people in general: be your real self because life is short. Own yourself and learn how to simply be because it just might be beautiful. Don't fear change or emotions, that's part of life and if you close out the scary parts, you'll close out the good ones with them. Don't fear the deep or the real. The worst that could happen is you'd meet yourself, and that could be the best friend you've been waiting for.

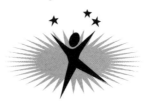

Accepting the Gift of Life

Lisa and Mike Sherman

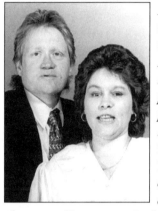

Lisa and Mike Sherman are both permanently disabled from the complications of diabetes. Lisa is totally blind. Mike is legally blind, has had two kidney transplants, quadruple bypass surgery, and one of his toes amputated. Together they spend many hours every week volunteering time to TECH 2000: Michigan's Assistive Technology Project, helping hundreds of other people with disabilities to locate devices and services that will help them to live more independently. They also volunteer their time educating others about the great need for people to consider being organ donors.

"And you married him anyway?" There I was, twenty-three years old and a new bride. The question was asked by a stranger, who couldn't fathom the idea that I had married my husband knowing that he needed a kidney transplant. Little did any of us know, that was only the beginning.

Mike and I met in 1985 at the Michigan Rehabilitation Center for the Blind. I was twenty-one years old, he was thirty-one, and both of us had just lost different degrees of our eyesight as the result of diabetes. Mike is considered "legally blind," still having a little vision, but unable to drive a car, read a newspaper, or see at

211

twenty feet what most people can see from 1,200 feet away. I, on the other hand, am completely blind. Both of us wound up at the Rehab Center looking for a way to learn how to be blind and hoping for a way to regain some of the independence that we had lost along with our eyesight.

Blindness is only one of the complications of diabetes, an insidious disease that robs its victims of proper circulation. That circulation loss results in blindness, kidney failure, nerve disease (diabetic neuropathy), strokes, high blood pressure, amputation of limbs, and heart failure. Technically, diabetes is the body's inability to burn sugar in the bloodstream. The pancreas of a diabetic person doesn't produce insulin, a hormone normally found in the bloodstream of nondiabetic people that changes the sugar in the blood into energy. When diabetics eat any kind of food, it is turned into sugar that sits in our bloodstream. Without insulin, the blood becomes thick, like a sugary syrup, preventing proper circulation. This in turn leads to the clogging, scarring, and breakdown of veins and arteries. Daily injections of synthetic human insulin help to control blood sugar levels, but they are not a cure.

When you are a diabetic, you don't really care about the technical aspects of the disease. You only know that over the course of years your body is slowly deteriorating, being eaten away by time. This is graphic perhaps, but it is a critical point nonetheless. When diabetes begins, the victims don't look sick. They take shots of insulin every day but otherwise live very normal lives: they go to school, play sports, ride bikes, and perform all of the other normal activities of life.

Time, however, is a cruel enemy. The constant fluctuation of blood sugar, and even the by-products of the life-saving insulin itself, work away at the veins and arteries, which eventually break down, usually about fifteen years after diagnosis. Then the devastating effects of the disease begin. The public is not very aware of how lethal diabetes is. When a diabetic dies, the cause of death is never listed as "diabetes," instead kidney failure, cerebral hemorrhage, or heart failure is cited.

While Mike and I were both diagnosed with juvenile diabetes, we were diagnosed at different stages of life. I was only two years old, while Mike was sixteen. Thus, while he has very definite memories of life without diabetes, daily insulin shots, and dietary restrictions, I have none.

The actual diagnosis of our diabetes was also very different, yet strangely similar. As is typical of uncontrolled diabetes, each of us experienced frequent urination and constant thirst. Mike's parents were tipped off that something was wrong not only because of these symptoms, but because their child lost thirty pounds in just one month, and they could literally see the sugar caked around his mouth. My parent's clues included a twenty-three-month-old baby who couldn't be potty trained and who woke up from naps with urine literally running out of the crib. I was unable to make a two-mile car trip from home to Grandma's without crying for a drink of water.

Completely frustrated, my mom took me to the pediatrician and begged for some answers. Tests were taken, and on my second birthday (in 1965) the doctor called to tell my parents that I was a diabetic and needed to be hospitalized. Naively, or what she today calls stupidly, my mom told the doctor that she couldn't possibly hospitalize me on my birthday. Thus, not understanding the implications of uncontrolled diabetes, and not knowing that I could have died during the night, my parents admitted me to the hospital the day after I turned two. My life would never again be the same.

Mike has very definite memories of going to the doctor to be tested for diabetes. He had to drink several bottles of a sugary, cola-flavored solution called glucola, and his blood sugar was then checked. Because he liked pop so much, Mike thought the test would be a breeze. After his first bottle, though, he was disgusted by the taste and couldn't wait for the whole thing to be over! The year was 1969, and Mike remembers that when the doctor called with the news his mother cried, and he thought only that now he wouldn't have to go to Vietnam. Years later though, Mike would be fighting a completely different, far more personal war of his own.

Ironically, although Mike and I were diagnosed with diabetes four years apart, both of our mothers recall the doctors telling them that the cure for this disease was just a couple of years away. More than thirty years later, there is still no cure. I sometimes wonder if those doctors really believed that at the time, or if they knew what was in store for the children of our young parents but wanted to offer them some hope.

Today, at thirty-two, I am considered to be a very lucky diabetic. My disease has only left me with high blood pressure, anemia, some kidney damage, and totally blind. At forty-two, Mike has not been as lucky. Legally blind, he too has high blood pressure. Additionally, he has also spent two years on kidney dialysis, had two kidney transplants, two heart attacks, quadruple heart bypass surgery, and most recently the amputation of one of his big toes. A typical day for us involves monitoring of blood sugar, multiple insulin injections, a regimen of medications, monitoring of blood pressures, dietary restrictions, and a need for exercise. Some people may view these activities as restrictive and inconvenient, but we just view them as our way of life.

Despite our diabetes and its related complications, Mike and I have always believed that we have a life before us, not just to live, but to enjoy. Aside from spending a lot of time in hospitals, we also spend much of our time doing volunteer work, listening to books on tape, gardening, and learning to use a computer. We've taken exciting vacations where we've parasailed and gone deep sea fishing, and quieter ones where we just visit family. I enjoy refinishing small pieces of furniture while Mike tinkers with a variety of musical instruments. In essence, we try to spend as little time as possible dwelling on the difficult events in our lives and spend more time focusing on the positives.

Mike and I also maintain our own home. While I do most of the cooking and cleaning, Mike takes care of the yard, the garbage, the mail, and balancing the checkbook. Most people are usually shocked by that. They assume that because we are visually impaired, that we are also incapable of caring for ourselves. People don't realize that it can be done. With practice, most people can maneuver around their own home with their eyes closed. Given time, they could probably even figure out how to slice vegetables, clean the toilet, fry bacon, broil a steak, put on make up, and use a curling iron, vacuum, or do the laundry.

After leaving the Rehab Center for the Blind in the spring of 1985, Mike and I knew that we wanted to be married. We also knew that people, especially our families, were going to think we were crazy. At that point I had lost my eyesight and Mike was legally blind and had spent the past year battling neuropathy, a nerve disorder that resulted in his inability to walk for many months. But we knew that we were meant to be together, and the following spring we were married.

Our wedding was very traditional. A white dress, tuxedos, lots of bridesmaids and groomsmen, flowers, trumpets, and organ music, all in an old stone church, with a beautiful reception to follow. My parents gave us a day that fantasies are made of. One very special moment came when the carillon bells at the church began to ring. I had thought that the added expense of the bells would be too much to ask of my dad, but when my mom asked him about it, he responded, "She can't see any of her wedding, let's give her as much to hear as possible." We ended the celebrations with a honeymoon in Florida, and set out to begin our life together.

Mike and I also announced that we were going to enroll in college. We were young, bright, and needed challenges other than those presented by our physical limitations. Neither of us knew what we could do after that, what kind of employment opportunities would await us, or if we would even be physically able to work, but we had to do something. So we enrolled, me in introduction to psychology and Mike in introduction to mathematics. Thus began a seven-year academic odyssey.

Returning to school wasn't a difficult decision, it seemed to be the only path open to us at the time. Mike had always worked as a bartender, and I had worked as a receptionist. Neither were careers that were tailor-made for people without vision! It wasn't simply an issue of choosing new career paths. Entering college as "alternative students" was a personal challenge.

Thanks to some of our training at the Rehab Center for the Blind, we had at least an idea of how to take a class, but for the most part, it was all trial and error. Tape recording lectures was an effective way to capture information, but ineffective in terms of studying. Instead of listening to four-hour lectures again and again trying to memorize key points, we would condense the tapes. Thus a four-hour lecture tape became twelve minutes of study notes. While this process was very time consuming, it was also a very effective study tool.

Our next hurdle was how to read a textbook. This problem was solved in part by an organization called Recordings for the Blind, a nonprofit agency that provides textbooks on audiotape for visually impaired students of all ages.

Taking exams was another issue. Each professor was different. Some would read the exams themselves and record our answers, while others would have a proctor read the exam. Still others would put the exam on a tape and allow us to tape record our answers. Either way, Mike and I were insistent that we be given no breaks. It was important to us that we be able to compete fairly with our peers, and with each other.

Yet another issue was how to produce reports and papers. This proved to be a task that would have been impossible without the help of many people. First, we needed to go to the library and gather information. Then we had to find someone to take the time to read the information onto a tape. Mike and I had to listen to the material and construct a report on another tape, and finally, find someone to transcribe the report onto paper. The most difficult part of producing a research paper was never the material itself, but finding someone to do the initial reading and then transcribing the final report.

Finally, how to get to campus? Mike and I own our home, about nine miles from school. We also happen to live in a town where there is no public transportation. Taking a taxi wasn't feasible for us either, as a one-way trip would have been $13. As was true for every other aspect of our lives, our family and friends turned out to be our saving grace. Each semester began with a fairly frantic series of phone calls to see who was available when. Something almost always worked out. At one point we even met a retired couple who not only drove us to our classes most semesters, but have also become very dear friends.

Transportation remains our biggest challenge today. If not for the generosity of Mike's parents, his sisters, and many of our friends, things like doctor's appointments, going to school, grocery shopping, banking, and the hundreds of other things that people do every day would be an impossibility for us. Relying on family and friends for transportation isn't always easy. There are many times when we miss something as simple as going to the corner store for a bottle of pop. Or times when I'm in the middle of cooking supper and I can't run to the store for a last-minute ingredient. When put in perspective of the rest of our lives though, these are not very big issues. In the seven years that it took us to complete our degrees, a lack of transportation forced us to drop our classes only once, and always in the back of our minds was "Will we make it through this semester without Mike going into the hospital?" Occasionally, the answer was no.

Two semesters after we had begun classes, Mike's kidneys failed. A shunt was surgically placed into his forearm, and several weeks later he began dialysis treatments. For three months, three hours a day, three days a week, Mike went to our local hospital and was hooked to a machine that cleaned toxins from his blood. While it saved his life, it also left him fatigued, anemic, and constantly cold. We spent that winter with Mike sleeping sixteen hours a day, fully dressed, under many layers of blankets with the furnace running at about 85°, and me wearing shorts and tank tops! So much for Michigan winters.

I wasn't sure that we would be able to finish that particular semester. Mike was only occasionally able to attend classes, so I would take my tape recorder and record the lectures. Mike would listen to the lecture tapes, study from my notes, and show up on exam days. I learned a lot from him that semester. I was ready to drop our classes and just stay home and care for Mike. Despite our wonderful family and friends, those were very lonely months. Instead of withdrawing though, I drew from Mike's strength. Seeing his desire to have a life that held something other than hospitals and doctor's offices, I committed myself to that end. We completed that semester with the focus on our classes. Our lives had only been interrupted by these events, not consumed.

Other changes were occurring during those months. Mike's sister Tracy courageously volunteered to donate one of her kidneys to Mike, and compatibility testing began. The transplant team at the University of Michigan Hospital determined that they were a very good match, and on January 21, 1987, our family witnessed a truly amazing thing. The kidney of a sister was removed and transplanted into her brother.

Nine hours after the surgery had begun, the doctors came out to tell us that it had gone well. It was an emotional day for everyone, but I often think of what it must have been like for Mike and Tracy's parents to sit and pray that the lives of both of their children would be spared.

Five days after surgery, Tracy was discharged from the hospital without complication. Mike was not as lucky. When the kidney still didn't work after twenty days, Mike was taken back into surgery. Scar tissue had wrapped around his urethra and was preventing the kidney from working. Even though that was eventually corrected, his body began to reject the kidney. Massive amounts of antirejection drugs were given. Five weeks later, with the kidney saved, Mike was discharged.

The fight for life that Mike put up during those two months was amazing. Still in kidney failure and on dialysis, rejecting his transplant, Mike was given drugs that produced vomiting, diarrhea, a temperature of over 105°, and hallucinations. He was in a hospital bed fifty miles from home, worried about me, our cat and dog, the house, and wondering if it would ever end.

It was only with the help of our parents and a dedicated hospital staff that Mike and I made it through those eight and a half weeks. My mom came in from out of town to stay with me for some of that time. She drove the one-hundred-mile round trip every day so that Mike and I could be together. When she left town, Mike's parents took over without question. Every day one of them would pick me up and make that long trip.

The nurses soon got to know us, and one day the charge nurse said, "You kids have been separated long enough." She then made arrangements for Mike to be in a private room, brought in a cot, arranged for meals to be delivered for me, and made it possible for me to stay with Mike for a few days at a time. Another nurse brought us diet ginger ale to drink out of plastic champagne glasses so that we could toast our nine-month wedding anniversary. When Mike was sent home with a ten-inch, open incision across his belly, the surgical nurse taught me how to clean, pack, and dress that gaping wound. That was very important to me. I didn't want my blindness to impede my ability to care for Mike. In the end, those selfless and loving acts, especially that of Tracy, allowed the transplant to work, and saved Mike and me from years of the debilitating effects of dialysis.

Despite the interruptions, Mike and I finished our college education seven years after we began. We even completed classes like art appreciation, environmental science (where we walked through the bogs of a local nature reserve), and statistics. Mike and I graduated with honors from Oakland University with degrees in psychology. It was truly our proudest moment.

During our last semester Mike and I also took a technical plunge and bought a computer. It wasn't just any computer though, it was a talking computer. It is almost impossible to describe the difference that this amazing piece of technology has made in our life. It has provided me with freedom and independence that I had previously thought were lost to me. Yes, there are tape recorders, and a reading and writing technique for the blind called Braille, but neither are as fast or as efficient as the computer. When I type something or read something, a voice synthesizer that is hooked to our computer repeats what is on the screen. With the push of a button it will repeat my text letter by letter, word by word, sentence by sentence, line by line, or page by page. Can you imagine the freedom that this provides? I am now able to access my address book or recipes in seconds, write a letter to my nephews in Chicago, and serve as recording secretary for a local volunteer organization. During our school years, I was finally able to type my own research papers.

Giving ourselves the gift of a college education was the best thing Mike and I could have done. We began as frightened, unsure, blind students, and graduated with far more than an education and a diploma. College provided Mike and me with discipline, motivation, courage, confidence, and the knowledge that with commitment, we could achieve anything. Little did we know, those lessons would take us far. Although those few months on dialysis and the complications following Mike's kidney transplant were both difficult and frightening, the true test of our ability to cope would come after graduation.

Though not superstitious, Mike and I have learned not to repeat that old adage about being careful what you wish for because it might come true. Mike always used to comment that he hoped his transplant would last long enough for us to complete school. He wanted nothing to prevent us from reaching that goal.

We completed our last class in August 1992. In September we celebrated our commencement ceremonies, and in October Mike had another shunt placed in his arm and was back on dialysis. After five and a half years, the transplant was being rejected. It was a reeling blow. Gone were any ideas of employment or furthering our education. Mike was immediately worked up for a second transplant. This time, however, there would be no family donor. Mike was placed on a waiting list with 32,000 other people in the United States awaiting transplants. Every day that we waited, eight of those people died. We could only pray that Mike wouldn't be one of them.

Could either of us possibly have known how true our wedding vows would ring? As is probably true for most married couples, the meaning of the words "For better or for worse, for richer or for poorer, in sickness and in health, until you are parted by death" took shape. We were now measuring them against hours spent in surgery, in waiting rooms, in numbers of hospital meals eaten, and in countless brief moments in recovery rooms and intensive care units.

During his transplant work-up, Mike failed his stress

test. Was there a problem in his heart? A procedure called a cardiac catheterization was ordered. A small wire with a camera on the end was inserted into an artery at Mike's groin and run up into his heart. This allowed the cardiologist to check for blockage or damage. If Mike wanted a kidney transplant they had to know first if he would be able to survive the surgery, and the test had to be done. Unbelievably, at some point Mike had suffered a silent heart attack, a heart attack, that, for any number of reasons, is not felt by the patient and is often not detected until more extensive damage occurs. One artery was completely closed and four more were severely blocked.

It was a horrifying moment when the cardiologist came out and told us that Mike would need quadruple bypass surgery. I struggled to keep my composure while Mike's dad left the waiting room to call home with the news. Mike, on the other hand, was lying back in the recovery room, incredulous that after all he had been through, now he needed open-heart surgery.

Four days later we met with a heart surgeon. A week after that Mike was admitted to the hospital for the bypass surgery. Never ready to admit defeat, Mike and I were hesitant to discuss the implications of open heart surgery. We spent that week telling each other that this surgery would be just like all the others, a few days in the hospital and then some recovery at home. Neither one of us could bear to say that it was the heart and that there was so much more that could go wrong. On the night before surgery though, we walked the halls of the hospital. Just as we approached his room, where both of our families awaited our return, Mike quietly squeezed my hand and whispered, "You know if anything happens to me you have to take care of yourself." I squeezed his hand back and whispered, "I know, I will." That was all we needed to say. We were determined that this surgery would go smoothly, and that was all the room we could allow for the possibility of death.

The next day, after seven hours of surgery, the surgeon came to tell us that Mike had done far better than he had expected. I'll never forget his compassion as he stood telling us about Mike, while gently rubbing my arm. He was a very caring man who seemed to realize that I was missing the reassurance of the eye contact that he gave to the rest of the family.

Mike called me from his bed in the intensive care unit the morning after surgery. I was shocked. The doctor had just told us that he might not wake up for a day or two, and here he was requesting his watch and his dentures.

The next day Mike was moved from ICU to a regular floor. We were on cloud nine. Gone were most of the wires and leads and tubes. Mike was recovering far faster than anyone expected, and it looked like clear sailing. Nothing is ever that easy though.

On the afternoon that Mike was moved out of ICU, my mom and I were at the hospital visiting. Mike was sitting up in a chair enjoying his lunch, and I was next to him, sitting on the bed, drinking the coffee that came on his tray. Mike suddenly got very quiet, and my mom softly called his name. Not being able to see what was going on, I asked if he was all right. My mom said that it looked like he was going into insulin shock, and ran for a nurse. The next fifteen minutes proved to be the most frightening moments of my life.

As my mom ran to get a nurse, Mike began gasping and choking for air. He was making the most unearthly sound I had ever heard. I couldn't do anything but scream for help. This was not insulin shock. As a nurse came running in, I did my best to move away from Mike, knowing that I would only be in the way.

A hundred things started happening all at once. My mom drew me out into the hallway as the nurse with Mike yelled, "We're calling a code." Suddenly an alarm started sounding throughout the hospital. A voice on the overhead intercom began repeating, "CPR team, room 7263, CPR team, room 7263." What sounded like a thousand people began running toward Mike's room. Mike was pulled from his chair, laid on the floor, and the nurses began resuscitation. I was literally paralyzed. I just stood there with my face buried against my mom. I couldn't even cry. I just kept shaking my head, and repeating, "No, no, no." The next thing I knew, the hospital chaplain appeared, and led me down the hall to a private lounge. There we sat for what seemed like hours, but was actually only about five or ten minutes. I had worked in a hospital for a brief time, and knew what it meant when a chaplain was summoned. Part of me was in shock, denying the whole experience. Another part of me was wondering what I was going to do when they came in and told me that Mike was dead.

A few minutes later Mike's surgeon and a few nurses came into the lounge. Mike was all right. They had gotten to him in time. The nurse who had reached him first took me by the arm and led me back to Mike's room. As we walked she kept rubbing my back and saying, "He's okay, we got him." Not realizing how intense the situation had been, Mike kept saying that he was embarrassed that he had caused such a fuss. The doctor couldn't explain what had happened, only that Mike had stopped breathing for a short time and needed to be resuscitated. For the next few days, Mike continued to have brief moments where he would pass out, but he al-

ways came around when we called his name. We never
had to go through the trauma of a code again.

Experiencing Mike's code and resuscitation by the
CPR team was a remarkable moment for me. Words
can't express how those few minutes changed my life. I
had just watched the most important person in the
world to me die and come back. While I had always
taken our marriage very seriously, I now had new perspective. Mike's courage during all of his surgeries, but
especially during the years of dialysis, were inspiring. I
would be damned if I would lose him now.

With the bypass surgery successfully completed, the
cardiologist could now declare Mike's heart strong enough
to survive kidney transplant surgery. On February 10,
1993, Mike was officially placed on the transplant waiting
list. At that time the wait for a kidney in the state of
Michigan was about three years, and the whole bypass experience had set us back almost five months. Mike was not
doing very well on dialysis. The rigors of removing his
blood three times a week, cleansing it, and then putting it
back in his body were taking their toll.

More and more Mike and I began functioning like
one person. Mike's energy was focused on the physical
side of his disease, willing himself to stay strong enough
to receive a transplant. I was focused on keeping us in-
tact both physically and emotionally. I could only
imagine how it must be to be so weak and tired and
dizzy that getting a drink of water was a challenge.
Every bump and sound took on new meaning. Was it
Mike passing out again? There were times when I truly
felt that I was living on the edge. Would I get to him in
time if he fell? Would his potassium get too high and
stop his heart? I even felt afraid to fall asleep at night
because I might not hear him if he needed help.

Our lives became very quiet and began to revolve around dialysis. The ambulance would pick Mike up, he would spend about four hours at the hospital, come home and sleep for most of the day, and then lie down most of the evening because he was too dizzy to sit up. Those years also showed me how strong I could be. It's funny though, I balked at letting Mike see how well I could manage alone; I didn't want him to get the idea that I could make it without him!

Something had to change. We knew that if we let it, the effects of life on dialysis would consume us. Ten months after starting dialysis, and seven months after going on the transplant waiting list, Mike and I realized that we were far from being defeated. We heard about a local clinic that devoted its time to helping people who had suffered vision loss, and wondered if we might not be able to help. We had each suffered a degree of blindness, and hoped that we might be able to help someone else to adjust. We started by going in once a week and making phone calls to clinic patients. The calls were a kind of support group. We had already gone through many of the things that these patients were afraid of, and oftentimes we were able to reassure them.

After a while, Mike and I started facilitating support groups, and helping out however we could. Mike would sometimes make telephone support calls from home, and I helped the director set up a Christmas shopping trip for the patients. It made us feel good that we could help others after so many people had helped us. We knew that there was no way to properly thank Mike's parents for all the driving they did for us, or to thank our friends and other family members who had helped us so often. The only thing we could do was to pass the kindness on, and help someone else.

Eventually the rigors of dialysis became too much for Mike and we found that we had to discontinue our volunteer work for a while. It was now the spring of 1994, and Mike had been waiting for a kidney for over a year. The average wait was about three years, and we weren't sure Mike could make it that long.

Along with our other volunteer work, I also began an organ donor awareness campaign. Mike was deteriorating before my eyes and I felt that I had to do something. The more I learned, the more horrified I became. Not only were more than 32,000 people waiting for transplants in the United States, and eight of those people died every day while they waited, but of the 15,000 people who died in the United States every year in circumstances that would allow them to donate their organs, only 4,500 actually donated. Translated, those numbers meant that if every person who could donate their organs actually did, there would be no organ waiting list. People waiting for transplants would stop dying at such an alarming rate.

I began my organ donor awareness campaign by writing a chain letter to 200 people. I told them about the need for organ donation, and asked them to pass the information on to five more people. I then began contacting the media, writing letters that pleaded for television shows and newspapers to do stories on organ donation. I received calls for more information from Erin Moriarty of "48 Hours," and Deborah Norville of CBS. A local Detroit newspaper even wrote about our awareness project. I then began contacting local libraries, shopping malls, schools, and bars asking them to place information about organ donation in their facilities. Everyone was interested, and once they understood our personal situation, they were very eager to help. One local company, Hussman Econometrics, paid for the printing of 2,000 informative newsletters. Another company called Advanced Automotive paid for information sheets to be printed.

My next project was to write to every professional baseball, football, basketball, and hockey team in the United States. I told them about our personal situation and the need for organ donor awareness, and asked that they consider having an organ donor awareness day in their ballparks and stadiums. Again, another local company, the Alexander Hamilton Insurance Company, stepped in and paid for the postage for these hundreds of letters to be mailed. A couple of teams picked up on the idea and held such days. Now, with the help of the Mickey Mantle Foundation, every major league baseball park in the country will have an organ donor awareness day.

I was feeling almost frantic. Not only was Mike still waiting, but friends that we had made through dialysis were starting to die. I contacted our local city council and asked them to announce Organ Donor Awareness Week (in April) on the televised city council meeting. They went a step further and had a plaque made that declared it was Organ Donor Awareness Week in Rochester Hills, Michigan. Eventually, I even began making presentations on the subject to local service clubs. People were dying needlessly because of a lack of education, and I didn't want Mike to be one of them.

The kindness of people amazed me—not only the people in my own community, but those from outside the community. My family in Chicago and New York helped by distributing newsletters in their churches. Hearing of our plight, a member of my sister's church asked for our address and sent us a check for $100 so that we could continue to print our newsletter. Mike and I were so touched by that gesture that we promised her we would find a way to pay a similar kindness to someone else.

On June 1, 1994, our prayers were answered. Mike was getting ready for dialysis, and I happened to be sitting by the phone. When it rang, I could not have been less prepared for what I heard. It was Carolyn from the transplant center telling me that they had a kidney for Mike. This was a call that we had waited almost two years for, and it was a complete shock when we finally got it! After almost two years, the wait was finally over.

I immediately sent out a prayer for the family who during a time of incredible grief had made a decision that would save the lives of seven people and give sight to two more. Mike's donor was a forty-year-old gunshot victim. People asked us whether he was the good guy or the bad guy, and we respond that whatever he was in his life, he was a hero in his death. Although we will never meet the family that made that incredible decision, we continue to thank them in our thoughts and prayers, and hope that the knowledge that their generosity gave life to so many people gives them some degree of peace. They too are heroes.

Mike was wheeled in to surgery at 10 o'clock that night. His mom and dad and I sat down to wait. By 2 A.M. we were the only ones left in the waiting room, and began forming makeshift beds out of chairs and blankets. When the surgeon finally came out at 6 A.M., he informed us that the transplant had gone well, and Mike would be moved up to the intensive care unit.

Nine days after surgery, Mike was doing well and was released from the hospital. Ten days later, however, his blood work came back abnormal and he was readmitted. Mike's body was rejecting the transplant. Again, he was given a series of massive antirejection drugs that made him very ill. At one point his electrolytes were so far from normal the doctors worried that his heart would stop. The treatment appeared to have worked though, and two weeks later, Mike was once again sent home.

Mike was feeling wonderful, and I was relieved to have him home. Seven days after he was discharged, we began volunteering again. This time, however, we decided to donate our time to a local community service council. Through a grant from TECH 2000: Michigan's Assistive Technology Project, our local Lions Club and the Rochester Hills Public Library set up a council to provide information about assistive technology services, devices, and funding sources for people with disabilities. The project seemed tailor-made for both of us. I was asked to be the council secretary, and Mike was asked to be the data entry coordinator for the Michigan Assistive Technology Clearinghouse (MATCH), a database of resources for the disabled.

Joining the TECH 2000 council was a true turning point for us. Mike had been so sick for so long, and we weren't sure what direction our lives were going in. I had often begun to think that our only role in life was to be professional patients. TECH 2000 offered us an alternative. As Mike puts it, "I was just happy to be a part of something." Coupled with the fact that this was going to provide us the opportunity to serve people with disabilities, we were very honored to participate.

Two weeks after our first council meeting, Mike developed a high fever. In a matter of hours, he had gone from being full of energy to a man who could barely function. Mike was in rejection. His body was rejecting the very transplant that was designed to save his life. For the third time that summer Mike was admitted to the transplant unit at William Beaumont Hospital. He had already run the gamut of antirejection drugs and there was little they could do for him except give massive doses of steroids and put him on an experimental immunosuppresent. The new drug appeared to work. Approved for liver transplants, the Food and Drug Administration had not yet approved FK506 for use in kidney transplants. It was, however, Mike's only hope.

The new immunosuppresent started working, and Mike's body began accepting the transplanted kidney. More than a year has passed since that time, and the kidney continues to function beautifully. Mike is happy, energetic, and if you ask him how the transplant makes him feel, he responds, "I feel alive for the first time in three years."

Our experiences with being on the transplant waiting list, and the transplant itself, taught us many things. First and foremost, we learned that we took Mike's first transplant for granted. He was sick and dying, and his sister was there without hesitation to offer him a second chance at life. It wasn't that easy the second time around though. There would be a long wait, and people we knew died while they waited. With the knowledge that we gained from the second transplant, we felt obligated to educate others. If our experience educates just one person, and that person makes the decision to be an organ donor, that's seven more lives that are saved, two people who are given the gift of sight, and dozens of accident and burn victims who are given skin grafts, bone grafts, and new ligaments and tendons. We have also learned a great deal about speaking out for things that we believe in. People who are not directly affected by organ transplants don't know what a difference they can make in someone's life. They see only the negative media stories about celebrity status and an unfair system.

While I do not deny that those are potential problems, I can only encourage people to look at our story and see a family that was in desperate need and the heroic efforts of another family who made the decision to give us life again. And don't forget the thousands of success stories that you don't see on the nightly news.

Most important, Mike and I have learned about ourselves. Not only with this last transplant, but with our entire lives, we have learned what we mean to each other, and what we can offer to others. Mike is a man who has accepted his life with courage and dignity, and has taught me to do the same.

Never relishing the thought of another medical complication, Mike always accepts each crisis with a "let's do it and get it over with" attitude. He has devoted himself to our life together, and learned that I am devoted to the same. I was so touched once to hear him describe me as "never being discouraged by what goes on in our lives." He went on to praise my "never wavering love," saying I have given him "more than any other person possibly has, or could have." I can only respond by saying that that's what you do when you love someone. Mike and I learned at a very early age that our lives will be shorter than most, and that we need to make the most of what we are given.

After his last discharge from the transplant unit, Mike and I returned to our volunteer work with TECH 2000. The project has provided us a great opportunity for personal growth. Though not paid positions, Mike and I feel very proud of the work we do. Diabetes has wrought great havoc in our lives, but we can now take those events and turn them into something productive. Individually, and as a couple, we have been through the proverbial wringer, and have a lifetime of experiences to share with others. If nothing else, we hope that our experiences can provide motivation and hope for someone else.

As a council we have accomplished incredible things, and Mike and I are proud to be a part of it. Nothing can compare with the feeling we got from helping a twelve-year-old blind boy to get a voice synthesizer for his computer, so he can now play computer games just like other children; or the woman with cerebral palsy who received a donated computer from the council and has since set up a typing service out of her home. Perhaps most rewarding was an eleven-year-old visually impaired child who had become withdrawn. He was failing school and didn't want to socialize with other kids. The council arranged for his textbooks to be copied in large print and located a closed circuit TV that would enlarge his homework. This boy is now bringing home straight A's and playing baseball with other children.

We're also involved in more comprehensive projects. When a local van company that serves seniors and the disabled attempted to violate the Americans with Disabilities Act by charging handicapped riders more than the seniors, Mike and I became involved and had the policy reversed. We've also started a letter-writing campaign designed to bring the Americans with Disabilities Channel to our local cable system. Recently we began assisting with a council project that collects donated computers that are refurbished and given to people with disabilities so that they can join the information superhighway. Mike and I get a thrill knowing that our efforts are helping others.

My talking computer allows me to keep meeting minutes, correspond with scheduled speakers, research resource information, and assist Mike with data entry. Mike's primary role is to locate information about assistive technology services, devices, and funding sources. He then verifies the information and enters it into the statewide MATCH database. We also speak publicly and do individual investigations into resources for people. This rewarding work takes little more than twenty hours out of our week, but those are twenty hours when Mike and I feel like whole, productive, meaningful, contributing members of society. We continue to say that this project gives us far more than we give it. We were honored to be named the 1996 TECH 2000 Volunteers of the Year, but feel that the true reward comes from knowing that we have helped someone else.

As is true for everyone, we never know what is around the corner. Just last month Mike developed an infection in his foot, and had to have one of his big toes amputated. When we come across challenges, people ask how we cope with all that has happened to us and how we continue to cope. The answer is simple but not easy. Mike and I can cope because to us, our life is what it is. While I wouldn't go as far as describing it as normal, it is what we were given. Now it is up to us to make the best of it. If we fell apart every time we came up against something difficult, our whole lives would fall apart. It's that simple.

With the legacy of this devastating disease never far away, Mike and I are determined to take what we've learned and help others. Our lives are affected by diabetes and its complications, but they are not consumed by it. Every milestone in the last ten years, whether physical or emotional, has brought us to this point. We firmly believe that helping others and a commitment to the life and time that we have been blessed with is the only effective way that we can repay everything that has been done for us.

Mike and I are determined to keep living, to keep fighting this disease, and to keep our situation in perspective. While we certainly wouldn't have chosen to have diabetes and its complications, that's the reality of our situation. Instead, we realize what life has given us, accept it without surrendering to it, continue to live the best life that we possibly can, and encourage others to do the same.

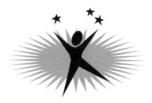

Author's note: On August 31, 1997, Mike suffered a sudden heart attack. Three days later, I sat holding his hand and his family gathered around his bedside as Mike was taken off life support. He died peacefully, his long and courageous battle with diabetes over.

The week before he died, Mike was busy obtaining donated computers so people with disabilities could access the information superhighway. He was enrolled in a computer class at our local community college and had just completed a letter-writing campaign to promote a local disabilities awareness project. It is my hope that others will learn from the example that Mike made of his life: Never give up, never lose hope, and never stop asking what you can do for someone else.

Coping, Caring, Creating, Conquering

Jean Griswold

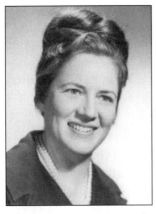

Jean Griswold has had multiple sclerosis for thirty years and is confined to a wheelchair. Fifteen years ago she founded Special Care, now a multi-million dollar company that provides home health-care services for the elderly, the disabled, and children with special needs. She has forty-two offices in seven states, employs more than 5,000 people, and is has been listed in both Who's Who in U.S. Executives *and* Who's Who in Professional and Executive Women. *Griswold charges clients less than other sources of such help and pays her employees more. She puts the company's profits into her nonprofit Special Care Foundation to pay for people who otherwise could not afford Special Care. Jean and Special Care have been featured in* Forbes *and* Entrepreneur *and on the "Today" show, among other places, and in 1996 Jean was named one of Pennsylvania's fifty "Best Women in Business."*

Multiple sclerosis (MS) hit me out of the blue. When the strange symptoms that had plagued me for several years (numbness, loss of balance, acute pain) were finally diagnosed as MS in 1969, I was determined not to let it hold me back. I managed to maintain pretty much the same hectic pace I always had. Only when we visited my son at the University of

Virginia and I was barely able to climb the long steps into the football stadium, did I finally have to admit that I was suffering from an insidious disease I could not overcome through sheer will power.

When our old family doctor made a house call to tell me that I had MS, he brought with him his ancient little black bag. From it, instead of a stethoscope, he produced an orchid to soften the bad news. I had no idea of the impact it would have on my life or why he warned, "Don't go look it up in the dictionary," although I now have a pretty good idea of both.

Multiple sclerosis is a totally unpredictable disease of the brain and nervous system. For reasons that are not yet fully understood, the material that insulates the nerves is attacked by the body's immune system and destroyed. Plaque forms where the damage occurs and interrupts the nerves' ability to transmit messages, resulting in a loss of feeling and/or motor control. Almost any function in the body can be affected, depending on which nerves become damaged. Numbness in the extremities, acute pain, and periodic episodes of fatigue are common symptoms, as are loss of coordination, balance, and bladder control. In more advanced cases, paralysis, permanent blindness, or even death may result. There is no way to predict how quickly MS may progress, what symptoms may be experienced, and which symptoms will be permanent.

Because the symptoms of MS may mimic virtually any other disease, until recently diagnosis has been very difficult and usually arrived at only by a lengthy process of elimination. Now, however, procedures like MRIs (magnetic resonance imaging) and CAT scans make diagnosis much easier and more definitive. Little progress has been made, though, in reversing the disease or controlling the symptoms.

My MS flared up at scattered times, but my life was so busy I felt I didn't have time to let it lay me low—physically or emotionally. I truly thrive on challenges and like trying to beat the odds. I like proving that I can accomplish things. As my MS has worsened over the thirty years that I have had it, each new set of symptoms demanded creative changes in my living environment and in my social and professional life. For a while I tried to cover up my symptoms, even though my bouts of dizziness while I was walking and stumbling gait sometimes made me look like I was drunk. I avoided walking where people could watch and stare. I changed my ideas of what I had to do. I coped without paying much attention to my increasing handicaps.

I have always liked to work, so I decided to get a full-time job as my sons grew and left home for college. I applied for an exciting management-level job and was on the verge of being hired when my best friend, whose name I had given as a reference, commented to my prospective employer, "She'll do just fine, even with her MS." It was the kiss of death!

As *Entrepreneur* magazine wrote in their July 1991 issue, "She couldn't get a job, so she created one."* Fifteen years ago I founded what has become a multimillion-dollar home health-care company with forty-two offices in seven states. I wasn't about to let multiple sclerosis stop me from being productive.

Being a very busy, active person, I found it hard not being able to always go where I wanted and needed to go. I cannot walk at all, and cannot transfer myself into and out of my wheelchair without the assistance of a me-

---

*Catherine O'Shea, "Never Say Never," *Entrepreneur* 19, no. 7 (July 1991): 180–85.

chanical lift and someone to operate it. I have learned to use the telephone to invite colleagues and competitors to come to my office to meet with me. I have used my wheelchair, at first hesitantly, then with adventure, to get to affairs and to appear on stage when I am asked to speak or receive an award. Yes, it's embarrassing, mostly because it's awkward. I cause the planners of big events where I am being honored a lot of trouble. They have to set up a ramp to get me on and off the stage, and a microphone at wheelchair height. I have to wear long skirts to cover my legs, which are right at eye-level when I am sitting on stage. I want people to be able to focus on my message and my business rather than on my illness and its attendant problems.

I began Special Care because a widow in the church of which my husband was the minister wanted someone to stay with her at night. She was lonely and afraid. Even though she could afford to hire someone, she was unable to find an appropriate companion. She neglected herself, was hospitalized, and died. When I learned the details, I became convinced the tragedy could have been prevented. The right kind of help would have saved her life. I was determined to use my education and professional experience in counseling to do something. I began to gather a pool of carefully screened, intelligent, caring people who were willing and able to serve as part of what was first known as Overnight Sitting Service and later as Special Care.

I started the organization at my dining room table. As more and more calls came in from people in the area who desperately needed help, I began adding case workers to match up the needs and the available personnel. Special Care took over the living room, and then a newly-enclosed porch as the pool of compassionate moonlighting seminary students was enlarged to include hundreds of trained nurses' aides available twenty-four hours a day.

The growing elderly population was waiting. I just had to make sure the quality of our nurses' aides was always given top priority. I could never forget that my reason for working seven days a week, twenty-four hours a day was to help people. The fact that I was also making money really surprised me.*

Much of my time was spent finding the kindest, most reliable, and intelligent aides to go out into homes, to fix a meal, give a bath, help with pill-taking, write a letter, take someone to the doctor, pull on stockings and shoes, brush teeth, comb hair, do some laundry, or even change a burned-out light bulb.

My theory has always been to try to find caregivers who live as close to their patients as possible so that they can reach the the patients even in heavy rain or snow, whether at 6 A.M. or midnight, and so they are familiar with the neighborhood stores for shopping or outings. I began licensing other highly motivated people to launch clone operations in manageable exclusive territories. Now we have seventeen offices in Pennsylvania and another twenty-three ranging from Boston to Key West.

When the township told me to "cease and desist" because I was operating a business in a residentially

---

*Clients of Special Care pay their nurses and companions directly, but they do pay a registry fee to the company, and although Special Care is a "for profit" company, we usually say it's a "lean profit company," as we have tried to keep the overhead as low as possible so that the registry fee remains low. For those who really cannot afford even the low rates charged by Special Care, the Special Care Fund has been established and it has thus far provided over $80,000 in subsidized care.

zoned neighborhood, I thought Special Care was finished. I could no longer walk or drive. If I could no longer have my business in my home, how would I be able to get to work? I persuaded the township to give me time to locate an office building, sell my home, and move into an apartment over the Special Care office. At first I used a stair-guide to get between floors; then, when I could no longer transfer out of my wheelchair, an elevator became necessary for the trip from my bedroom to my office.

As the founder of a successful company, I was written about, interviewed, televised, and turned inside out for unique personal stories. It's a hassle. It's an honor. Meantime, I have many demands as a chief executive officer. I must read widely and study to be informed and alert to federal and state regulations and to keep current on effective business practices. I need to know and understand how to use new equipment and business tools—copiers, computers, voice mail, fax—both to make my business more efficient and to enable me to compensate for my challenged physical condition. I have always been reluctant to talk about my MS—I believe it is a waste of other people's time and of mine. I prefer to focus on Special Care. It is my business that matters, not my condition. Special Care has become my life. I love it.

Starting a business is like a disease. You catch the idea and it permeates your whole system. You begin to spend day and night planning and networking. Women who are good have an edge. They are fascinating, driven, and intriguing. I used to think I had to use a powerful, commanding voice to sound serious and important. Now I believe my appeal lies in being very feminine and sweet, coupled with an overdose of intelligence and skill.

Special Care saves lives. Everybody needs somebody, if only to do the little things like picking up a pair of glasses that dropped on the floor just out of reach. Special Care enables people to remain living at home where they can hear the neighborhood children, watch their favorite TV programs, and eat their favorite foods, even in their failing years. It shelters people from the feeling that life is over, that they've made their last move to a nursing home, where cries of "Take me home" fill the ears of visitors. It lets them stay in their comfy, old, four-poster bed amid their memories.

The many awards that I have received please me, not because of the honor, but because I want my life to count for something. On my wall hangs a plaque that reads:

> I expect to pass through this life but once.
> If therefore there is any kindness I can show,
> or any good I can do to any fellow being,
> Let me do it now.
> Let me not defer or neglect it,
> For I shall not pass this way again.
>
> A. B. Hegeman

The real reward that I have received from Special Care has not been the notoriety gained from being featured on the "Today" show, or in *Forbes* and *Entrepreneur* magazines, but the satisfaction of knowing how much others have benefited from the services—the essential physical support for a bed-bound individual and the equally essential emotional support for an exhausted spouse—that Special Care provides.

The Spirit of Philadelphia award that I received in October 1988 warms my heart with its affirmation: "Your caring and unselfish commitment of time and en-

ergy set an example for all of us." Each time I look at the
plaque with its bronze Liberty Bell I remember how surprised I was when WCAU-TV Channel 10's anchor news
reporter, Alan Frio, arrived at my office with camera
and sound crews to present the award and to interview
me for the broadcast. Such recognition from the public
media gave me a welcome validation that what I was
doing through Special Care was indeed significant
enough to be newsworthy.

Apart from bureaucracy-plagued Medicaid and/or
welfare, there are very few places where poor, disabled,
and elderly people can get the help they need but can't
afford. For a number of years now, Special Care has contributed a portion of its profits to the Special Care Fund,
which pays part or all of the cost of care—at least until
some other "safety-net" can be found—for desperately
needy individuals who literally have no place else to
turn. Support for the Special Care Fund has increasingly been coming from families who are grateful for the
dedicated, loving care their dying mother or father or
child received from Special Care caregivers.

I sometimes wish I could get out of my wheelchair so
I could give a hug to each of the wonderful, faithful
nurses' aides who don't hesitate to go out in pouring rain
at ten o'clock at night to be with their dying patient and
to assure their patient's family that there is someone
there who understands and cares and can help with the
stages of dying. Few people realize how tough it is to
drop one's personal life and devote time and energies to
the unpleasant and all too often unappreciated aspects
of caring for the sick, the infirm, and the dying.

I value the little things that help me cope: being
pushed close to my office desk, my feet propped on a
cushion hidden under my desk, my phone within reach

and my outgoing mail given to the mail carrier; my staff refraining from asking every day, "How are you?" because they know I don't want to waste time talking about me when there are crises to handle and care to arrange for; and other similar, ordinary comforts. Even more, I value big things, like friends who really understand the daily struggle and stay friends, even when I can't do things for them. They are precious friends indeed.

I value the gift of patience that enables me to wait when I'd rather be doing, and to be able, when the mind is willing but the body is too weak, to accept the well-intended remarks of people who say, "Well, you look fine, so why can't you come?"

I value my three sons, each of whom has taken the time to build a ramp for my wheelchair so I can get into his home and is more than ready to drop everything in order to help push me up that ramp.

I need more time to do the same amount of work, since everything takes me twice as long to do as it would an able-bodied individual. Even getting dressed to go to work each morning is like putting in a full day's work. Multiple sclerosis causes overwhelming fatigue to set in after half a day's work, but I need, and want, to work all day long. Sitting in a wheelchair, even when made as comfortable as it can be, wears down one's resistance to pain. There is an urgent need to move around at least a little, but the paralysis caused by the MS makes it impossible.

I live for my work and see no future apart from it, because it is the vehicle through which I can share, care, and love not only the lovable but also those who need love most desperately. That's why I make plans for the future. Each day is a gift. My job each night is to plan carefully what I still need and want to do and to schedule what and when I can fit it in. My long-term plans also focus on my work, because I love and live my work. It keeps me alive and interested, financially, personally, and professionally.

My advice to others is to find someone or something to love. It is in giving that you receive. No matter what adversity or handicap may come your way, if you have love, there are always new and creative ways to make your life count.

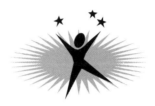

The Climb of My Life

Laura Evans

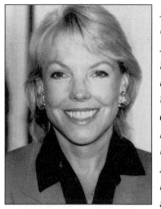

Laura Evans was diagnosed with breast cancer at the age of thirty-nine. In 1993 she founded Expedition Inspiration, a nonprofit organization that lends support to breast cancer survivors and helps raise funds to find a cure for the disease. In 1995 she helped lead a courageous team of breast cancer survivors to the top of Mt. Aconcagua in Argentina, the highest peak in the Western Hemisphere, to raise awareness, hope, and funds for breast cancer research. Laura has been featured in many newspapers and magazines and has appeared on numerous national television and radio programs, and much of her time is spent giving motivational speeches.

I had only heard or, more correctly, registered the word "cancer" once before, when my grandmother was dying of it, slowly, painfully, and without hope. I had read the word many times, of course, in obituaries. Cancer, the death word.

I heard the word "cancer" again when I was diagnosed with it at the age of thirty-nine. I was too young to die—and too healthy—I thought. I had recently returned from an arduous trek in Nepal and felt rejuvenated physically and mentally. I felt stronger than I ever had in my life. I was incredulous to be told I had metas-

247

tasized breast cancer, cancer that had spread from my breast to my lymph system, and only a 15 percent chance of surviving the next three to five years. How could that be?

Until this time, I had never dealt with my own mortality, with our natural human fear of the reality of death. I thought I would continue to rock and roll my way through decades to come. In those dark moments during the diagnosis and subsequent treatment, I thought a lot about life and death. I also thought a lot about the quality of my life, pressures, and stress.

Before I became sick, I allowed myself to be swept up in a myriad of responsibilities, commitments, and hobbies; expecting far too much of myself. I never stopped to evaluate what I was doing. Was this working for me? Was I doing this for me or for someone else? Down deep, was I really happy? I left little time to dream. Now I would be fighting for my life. To increase my chances of long-term survival I opted for a clinical test which included seven weeks in a sterile hospital isolation cubicle undergoing intensive chemotherapy followed by a bone marrow transplant. It was a scary proposition. It was also desperately lonely being removed from any human contact, especially when I was sick and hurting, but it allowed me to focus all my energy on getting well. I visualized cancer cells being catapulted into the ocean and devoured by fish. I filled my mind and heart with what I perceived to be a healing white light. I looked out my window at the lush green park across from the hospital and vowed that one day I would walk through it. I dreamed of once again climbing mountains and I religiously crossed the days off my calendar one at a time.

I almost died in the hospital, feeling myself lifted gently into a quiet place, devoid of pain and suffering. I was drawn back to life by the faces of those friends and family staring through the clear vinyl bubble, anxiously hoping for my recovery. I never forgot that moment which erased my fear of death. I was left with the certain knowledge that death, when it came, would be a welcome release. I also knew, for the first time, that life doesn't have to be so difficult. We make it that way. It is important in life, as in death, to release the pain and suffering and focus on the joy.

When I left the hospital I was easier on myself, more accepting of who I was and of those around me. I also walked through that beautiful park. Because I had been denied being outdoors, my appreciation of nature intensified. The sky was bluer, the sound of the birds sweeter, and the mountains beckoning. I have always found solace in nature: the hills and trees and rivers seem to balance out any stress and confusion in my life. Now as I tried to put together the pieces of my life, I relied on that balance even more. As I wandered through the hills that embrace my hometown of Sun Valley, Idaho, I found myself dreaming, out loud, in the daytime.

After surviving my experience with cancer, I vowed to help others deal with the trauma of this disease. One feels so lost, so alone, and so frightened when diagnosed with cancer. I wanted to show others the face of a survivor, to say, "Yes, there is hope." Before I got sick, I had planned to climb Mt. Kilimanjaro in Africa. Because of the harshness of my treatment, it took two long years of building back for me to finally stand on that 19,340-foot summit. When I did, it was a tremendous affirmation of the body's ability to recover if the mind allows it to. The positive reaction to my climb up Kilimanjaro planted the seed to climb an even bigger mountain, with other breast cancer survivors, in order to raise awareness, funds, and hope.

One day I dreamed of starting Expedition Inspiration and I couldn't shake it. I have learned, often the hard way, to follow my instincts. I learned that only I know what is best for me. I also learned to listen to the signals, the energy waves that criss-cross our lives that we too often ignore. I pursued the idea of Expedition Inspiration, a climb up 23,000-foot Mt. Aconcagua in Argentina, the highest mountain in the Western Hemisphere, with other breast cancer survivors. I conceived the journey as a tribute to breast cancer survivors everywhere; a fact that would demonstrate that through positive attitude determination and will, one can live with a life-threatening illness and still go on to achieve unlimited goals. Also, by having breast cancer survivors climb one of the highest mountains in the world, we could call attention to the disease that had almost taken our lives. We set a fundraising goal of $2.3 million, $100 for each foot of the mountain.

The Aconcagua climb raised $2 million dollars for breast cancer research and an untold amount of awareness. Many people feel that no single project has done more for the breast cancer cause. Thousands of women and men gained strength from our efforts allowing them to better deal with surgery, chemotherapy, radiation, and the slow process of rejuvenating the mind and body. There are three more Expedition Inspiration climbs planned for 1997 and early 1998. These are Mt. Rainier in Washington, Mt. Vinson in Antarctica, and Mt. Aspiring in New Zealand. Through these and future climbs, as well as hikes and other outdoor events, we expect to raise millions more dollars for the cause.

Our first climb not only helped to raise awareness and funds, but it also changed the lives of those who participated. Ashley Summer Cox was one of the last climbers added to the Aconcagua team. I was very touched by her story. She was diagnosed with breast cancer at the age of eighteen during what should have been a routine breast reduction surgery. At such a young age, she was unable to find anyone to talk to or any support group where she felt she belonged. As part of the Expedition Inspiration team, she suddenly found herself surrounded by women of all ages who not only understood, but cared and shared her passion for the outdoors as well. There is no question that her involvement in the climb helped her move through this traumatic period and grow as an individual.

In the spring of 1995, about two weeks after the airing of a PBS documentary about the Expedition Inspiration Aconcagua climb, a middle-aged woman came up to me in tears. She told of her diagnosis and treatment and the frightening months during which she had battled the disease without the support of her husband, who steadfastly refused to talk about breast cancer. It wasn't until after he had seen the nationally aired documentary that he was able to understand and comfort her and openly discuss what she was going through.

After one of the premiere showings of the documentary, a young man in his early twenties approached me and vigorously shook my hand. He said, "I have never been sick a day in my life, but you have shown me that I can do whatever I set my mind to, that I can achieve things that I thought were out of my grasp. I thank you."

Author friends who felt my story should be told encouraged me to write my autobiography, *The Climb of My Life*.* From the response to the book I know that it has helped many people better understand the process

---

*San Francisco: Harper San Francisco, 1996.

of getting through a crisis and the realization that working through it takes time. The book has also made people recognize that what they are experiencing is not unique to them. They are not isolated. They are not the only ones to have ever felt the myriad of emotions associated with a potentially fatal illness. *The Climb of My Life* also underlines the importance of humor, support groups, and of evaluating one's life, thereby setting priorities that work best for each individual. My book is also a demonstration of setting goals and the ability to achieve them, even against great odds. It is a manual on how to follow your dreams.

A dear friend and neighbor, a young, attractive, athletic girl, was diagnosed with breast cancer following a routine mammogram. At a very fit thirty-five, she felt healthier than she ever had. The diagnosis was such a shock that she felt totally lost and confused. She broke up with her boyfriend, cut back on her training, and spent hours in tears. After she read *The Climb of My Life,* she approached me, gave me a hug, and told me that I had saved her life. She said, "I didn't know that this was a process, that everything I was feeling was a normal reaction. Now I understand the emotional imbalance I have been going through and can move on."

I am the founder, president, and chief executive officer of the Expedition Inspiration Fund for Breast Cancer Research, a nationally registered nonprofit charitable organization. In addition to running the foundation, I do a great deal of motivational speaking, which I enjoy. I have often felt that I am alive for a reason, and that reason, I believe, is to help guide and support others, to act as a role model to help others deal with adversity and lead more enriched lives. It is my goal to firmly establish annual Expedition Inspiration climbs, take A-level hikes, and organize other fundraisers throughout the country. I also want to ensure the future of our annual breast cancer symposium, a two-day conference that unites leading researchers to encourage the open exchange of the latest discoveries in order to accelerate the development of new and effective cancer treatments. I want Expedition Inspiration to reach a point where it is bringing in a minimum of a million dollars a year for research. Through the talents of our medical board and the findings of the symposium, we will be able to direct these funds to worthwhile projects that will hopefully stop the spread of breast cancer. Simultaneously, I want us to continue to help educate and support the many women and men whose lives have been disrupted by this insidious disease.

Personally, I intend to keep climbing for me and for others, as long as I am able. To quote our materials, "Until there is a cure, there is a climb."

I would advise women with breast cancer to educate themselves; find out what options are available to them; talk to different survivors, oncologists, and hospitals; and then make the decisions that work best for them. I would encourage them to take an active role in their treatment and to spend quiet time nurturing themselves. I think it is important for anyone going through a life-threatening illness to evaluate his or her lifestyle to determine what is and isn't working well and what could make him or her feel happier and more fulfilled.

Because of the overwhelming success of the initial Expedition Inspiration climb, my team members and I were honored at the White House in a private reception with First Lady Hillary Rodham Clinton. For my ongoing work, I was chosen as the recipient of the first ever Woman of the Year in Sports/Perseverance Award and was selected as a local hero in Idaho to carry the torch for the 1996 Olympic Games, held in Atlanta, Georgia. I received the Distinguished Alumna of the Year award from Stephens College in Columbia, Missouri, and was honored at the Duke University Comprehensive Cancer Center with the prestigious Jonquil Award, an award presented annually by Duke University to between one and three people who have made a substantial contribution to raising awareness and funds for the breast cancer cause. *The Climb of My Life* was nominated as a finalist in the motivational category of Books for a Better Life, the first annual self-improvement book awards established by the Multiple Sclerosis Society.

My one message to both people with disabilities and those who are able-bodied would be to live your life to the fullest. Dare, as I have, to dream out loud, and then follow those dreams. Start the day with a smile on your face because you are thrilled at what it may hold and end it with a smile because tomorrow will be another wonderful adventure. If in the process you can touch the lives of others, then all the better.

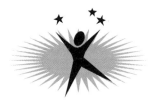

Following the Beat of a Different Drum

Evelyn Glennie

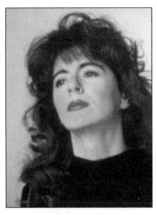

*Evelyn Glennie, thirty, has been pro-
foundly deaf since the age of twelve.
She is the first full-time solo percussionist in the world. She has played in
most of the world's greatest concert
halls, performing in over 120 concerts
every year and she recently released
her eighth CD. Two major documen-
taries on Evelyn's life have been made
for television and she has presented
and performed in two series of the
BBC's "Soundbites." Her exploratory
visit to Korea was the subject of a BBC television "Great Journeys" program. Her autobiography,* Good Vibrations, *was
published in 1990 (London: Hutchinson). Evelyn is the president of the London-based Beethoven Fund for Deaf Children,
a charitable organization that provides music-based therapy
for hearing-impaired children.*

> As a player I am in no man's land
> Let there not be war in music
> Music is circular like the shape of its notes
> Let there not be sides
> —Evelyn Glennie

For the first sixteen years of my life, our farm in
northeast Scotland, Hillhead of Ardo, known to the
locals less grandly as "Hillies," was the center of
our lives and each year followed the same pattern of

255

care for crops and animals. Fifteen years down the road, my mind often wanders back to my days on "the ranch," through season after season, looking after animals and land, and I reflect on the now-young hands of my oldest brother following in my father's footsteps. Despite all the many wonderful, exotic countries I have visited over the years, "Hillies" is undoubtedly my true home.

My musical upbringing was no more than the appreciation of Scottish traditional music and the sound of a tractor. No one quite knows where my enthusiasm for music came from. It didn't play an important role in either of my parents' lives while I was growing up. My mother enjoyed her organ playing and my father occasionally played the accordion. We had a piano at home but this was not pushed on me as something to pursue. My memory for little tunes was acute. One day I riveted everyone with a perfect rendering of the "Younger's Special" beer jingle from a television advertisement. The reaction was short-lived and "prodigy" and "genius" were, perhaps fortunately, not my family's immediate reactions. Music became increasingly important to me in a quiet and relaxed way and I was able to experiment and play the piano without external pressures.

My formal training on piano began at age eight. After attempts to play by ear the tunes and jingles that floated around the house from television, I was eager to learn more than my own tinkering could teach me. My mother arranged for me to have lessons locally. My piano teacher was a tall and strongly built woman in her sixties who had the misfortune of being extremely short-sighted. Her house was old and enormous, with a vast garden surrounded by trees. At the bottom of the garden she kept two magnificent peacocks. I loved to see them spread their tails to show off their brilliant feathers, stalking across the lawn with their crowns waving to and fro. One bright spot of my lessons, apart from chasing the pea-cocks to snatch a feather or two, was the was the arrival of a tray of biscuits (cookies) that was served while I waited for my friend to finish her piano lesson. Whoever had to wait first could enjoy seeing how many biscuits she was able to eat without the plate looking too empty. We both became extremely skillful at this!

In June 1974, when I was nine, I was entered for my first piano exam. I didn't bother to warm up before the exam, in fact, I have never practiced prior to any exams or auditions since. To this day I leave a gap between re-hearsals and concerts because I feel there is a greater spontaneity and freshness if I avoid the temptation of a last-minute rehearsal. At the sight of other candidates and their parents' long worried faces I thought we had arrived at our dentist's waiting room; the only difference was the jolly-looking staves and treble clefs that adorned the wall instead of diagrams of rotten teeth and fillings. The exam room was long, bare, and cold, with a piano at one end and a desk at the other. The examiner was, unusually for that time, a woman. It was probably even more unusual to have a candidate, me, who dic-tated which scales she wanted to play. I got away with this for the first two sets of scales, but then the exam-iner said gently, "Why don't you try D-major, right hand?" I always look people straight in the eye, which tends to give the feeling that I am totally committed to what is happening between me and the other person. With the examiner, it created a conversation between us rather than her just telling me to do this or that. Our time together ended with a bubbly "Cheerio" and "thank you." I went back to the waiting room with the proud feeling that I had met someone new without anyone else being there and for the first time had had a serious conversation solely about music. A week later I received the result. I achieved honors and the highest mark in the United Kingdom.

The immediate and exciting effect was that I was invited to give a short performance at Aberdeen's Cowdray Hall. This was the first musical milestone in my life. When my name was called to go on stage to play, I didn't hear it and the man behind me tapped me on the shoulder to take my cue. I climbed on stage and was faced with an enormous grand piano that had three pedals instead of the two I was used to. I didn't know which pedals to use. Everyone was looking at me, there on the platform for the first time in my life at age eight. I decided to launch in and make the best of the experience. When the audience applauded I had a terrific feeling of having all the attention to myself. I like being on the high stage looking down at all the faces, sharing something that excited me so much. I suppose this was the beginning of it all.

When I was ten I longed to play the clarinet, which I had picked out when watching orchestras on television. It had a warm velvety sound which I loved, and I was entranced by its slender and intricate appearance. My parents made a secret trip to Aberdeen to purchase the clarinet recommended by my teacher. I found it waiting for me one evening when I went to fetch the cutlery for the supper table: a beautiful shiny clarinet in a brand new black box. There was a finger chart in the back of my clarinet music book and, unknown to my teacher, I was soon busily exploring the chart so that I could try out my favorite pieces in the style of Acker Bilk, the famous clarinet player. My progress was healthy and after a few months I was attending a Saturday morning music school to play the clarinet and the recorder, another woodwind instrument.

For the next few years I progressed with the piano and passed seven of the eight exams with honors. I took my final exam at the exceptionally young age of fourteen. However, a serious challenge was forming. My hearing was so poor that my audiologist advised that instead of proceeding to a local comprehensive secondary school, I should attend the Aberdeen School for the Deaf. At age eleven I was looking at the prospect of being classified for life as disabled and cut off from the music that was beginning to seem vital to my happiness.

> So often we hear but don't cultivate listening
>   skills.
> Listening is cultivated inwardly when
>   your instrument can possess your whole being.
> It is this process that we can be frightened
>   of and intimidated by.

Growing deaf was such a gradual process that was many months before we realized that there was a serious problem. The first sign occurred when I was eight. I wrote in my little diary "I wonder if I am losing my hearing?" I began to have sore ears after riding my bicycle in windy weather and this progressed to the stage where I spent playtimes and breaks indoors at school to avoid going outside. I began to feel increasingly bewildered as things had to be repeated more and more. I didn't know whether I lacked ability in my classes or if I wasn't hearing clearly, but I was ready to explode. I knew I had so much room to grow and develop but I just wasn't getting anywhere. My mother eventually took me to our local doctor, who soon sent me to a specialist. Despite many, many tests in Aberdeen and Glasgow, no-body knew why the nerves in my ears had deteriorated. My mother eventually stopped my clarinet lessons be-cause she was worried about my ears, wondering whether the instrument and my efforts to play the high notes, which I did not yet have the skill to manage, were contributing to the loss of hearing.

To salvage what remained of my hearing, I began to wear hearing aids, causing quite a stir in our local area. It was unusual for anyone to have them, never mind an eleven-year-old child. My speaking voice grew higher in pitch. As sounds outside me got louder with the aids, I raised my voice to compensate. I grew to depend on the aids more and more. Unfortunately, the tiny batteries ran out at awkward moments. All my self-confidence disappeared when this happened.

I decided not to tell any teachers at my new compre-hensive school that I was deaf: I felt able to cope with the help of the hearing aids. My first real challenge came with a music test. Music was compulsory for the first-year pupils and we were given an aural test to dis-tinguish the musical students. We listened to a cassette tape asking questions and wrote our answers on a sheet of paper. I couldn't hear the tape properly—I only heard a horrible crackle. My spirits somehow were high even though the end result of the aural test meant that I scored the lowest mark in the whole year. I had already done well in my piano exams and was proficient on the recorder and clarinet. However, it was hard to convince the music teachers that I felt musical and that I wanted to try my hand at percussion.

After much pestering, I was finally given the chance to audition for a place to study percussion. It all went smoothly and my percussion teacher insisted he start teaching me immediately. I was conscious of my hearing aids and made sure my hair covered them. It wasn't until sometime later that I had my hair cut, allowing my aids to peep through slightly and become visible. From this moment on, the realization of my plight became apparent. The fact that I had appeared to be the most unmusical person in the world according to my aural test all made sense.

I went on wearing my hearing aids until I left school, but increasingly they became a waste of time. As a musician I found that I was improving with the mechanics of playing but everything else was out of control. I was losing my balance and coordination. Sounds were extremely distorted and it was increasingly difficult to identify where they came from. When I played in a group I could only hear noise and began to play louder and louder in order to hear myself—I couldn't relate to what my fellow musicians were doing. It was all very far removed from what I remembered as music, and I was so frustrated that I started to play with the volume turned down and eventually without using the aids at all.

To my surprise, I was no longer distracted by unidentifiable noise. I began to understand how to compensate for being deaf. I found I could control my movements so as to make soft or loud sounds, and I was beginning to recognize how much pressure I needed to strike a bar, and how the dynamics of a sound worked. The fact that I have perfect pitch, which means that I can hear the precise pitch of a note in my head and place it exactly in relation to other notes, has been a tremendous advantage. However, I did have problems tuning the timpani, a type of drum. These instruments have a pedal that can be raised or lowered in order to tighten or slacken the skin or head of the drum to adjust the pitch up or down. This is called pedal tuning. Hand-tuned timpani have several taps at the top of the drum which you turn to tighten or release the skin. I discovered that whichever drum I was working with, the slacker the skin the lower the note for that particular drum and the tighter the skin the higher the note. Because of my perfect pitch, I did, at least, know the notes to which I wanted to tune the drums and I learned to identify the different notes by the way in which my stick felt on the skin. If I played a low note the skin would be slack and my stick would stay on it longer. If the note was high the skin would be tight and the stick would bounce off immediately.

I can also tell the quality of a note by what I feel. My whole approach to holding my percussion sticks is different from most players, as I like to feel a sensation through the shafts of the mallets to my fingertips. My body is like a resonating chamber—highly alert to vibrations and impacts, dynamics, and all kinds of sensations. Over the years, my body has become highly tuned and sensitive, as is my concentration, focus, and commitment but most of all my imagination. I am like a child, I suppose, with nothing to prove in my playing as I constantly let my imagination run into overdrive—experimenting, falling and rising constantly.

> I wish you could hear the marimba of my imagination.
> It sounds so much better than the one you experience.
> I don't even play it with sticks.

One of the most beautiful aspects of percussion is that it is, I feel, the most social of all musical instruments. The young, old, rich, poor, professionals, beginners, ablebodied, and disabled can all participate in the playing of percussion. As I traveled, I realized that percussion is the backbone of many musical cultures such as Africa, Latin America, and Indonesia, among others. So often the spoken language can be a barrier but the drum is the true link. My curiosity toward this "social" aspect has led me to become an avid collector of old and new instruments with the extension of making my own. My collection thus far extends to over 700 instruments from all corners of the globe. My interest in percussion, interpreting both familiar and little-known instruments from every continent to musical audiences of all ages, has developed at a rapid rate.

My appreciation of Scottish traditional music has taken on a whole new and exciting dimension since my days on "the ranch" and now I am excitedly learning to play the Great Highland Bagpipes with the enthusiasm I had when I started studying percussion at the age of twelve. It is interesting to note that many of the great musicians I have worked with have, like me, spent hours, days, weeks, months, and years striving for perfection. Equally, I have collaborated with both professional and amateur musicians from India, Indonesia, Alaska, the Middle East, Korea, Ireland, and Scotland, to name just a few places. They can spend a lifetime specializing in one particular percussion instrument, such as the bodhran (a Celtic variation on the drum), marimba (a xylophone of southern Africa and Central America), tabla (a drum used in Indian music), snaredrum, or bones. They aim to become "one" with their instrument and find the crucial internal vibration that transfers them to a level or world that words cannot explain. Commercialism and technology are not usually a temptation to these musicians, and they guard their knowledge and discoveries fiercely.

On my travels, it has been vital to speak the same

raw musical language as my new musical friends, for they will only part with knowledge once they realize you are one of them. In fact, the balance I experience in "playing by ear" and digesting complex scores is a fascinating one and has led me to some of the most exciting times of my life.

My whole journey as a solo percussionist since the early days of my career has been truly exciting, dangerous, fascinating, frustrating, and many other things. I had the good fortune of progressing with music as a teenager at my own pace with no parental pressure. I had the feeling that music would always be a hobby and that my love of art would be my profession (it is now the other way around). Once I had decided, at the age of sixteen, to become a professional solo percussionist, I wasted no time or energy. I auditioned for two places only—the Royal College and the Royal Academy of Music, both in London. After enduring two auditions, on separate occasions, for the Academy (because they couldn't believe first time round that "a deaf musician could play so well"), I decided to accept the place at the Academy.

While my colleagues were deciding what to do with their lives within the field of music, I was determined and adamant that solo percussion would be my specialty. I graduated at age nineteen with an honor degree presented to me by Princess Diana. I studied both piano and percussion as joint first studies.* I gave the first solo percussion recital and concerto performances in the history of the Academy. I was the first deaf student to be accepted at a music institution in the United Kingdom and I started to be known as the first full-time solo percussionist in the

---

*"Joint first studies" is a designation akin to the American college term "double major."

world. Interestingly, the more I progressed the more I realized I was on my own. I had just assumed the world had other solo percussionists who traveled and worked in a similar way to a concert pianist or violinist. Perhaps my ignorance and naïveté have stood me in good stead.

I have had to work hard at many things over the years to sustain a career as a solo percussionist. In my early days as a performer I used violin, flute, and piano repertoire and arranged/transcribed them for percussion. Gradually I came into contact with composers who wrote pieces for me. Today the commissioning of concertos and recital pieces is one of the most important aspects of my work. You start with a seed; a piece grows, as do new techniques and instruments; the piece is performed, toured, and recorded; and then performed by other players. It is fascinating and satisfying to know that the piece has become part of the music world forever. I have at least ten new commissions in progress each year, which makes for a busy practice schedule in between approximately 120 concerts per year.

Another challenge is the equipment itself. I travel with over one ton of equipment, a large truck, a technician, and great stamina and patience. Percussion comes in all shapes and sizes which means the logistics of transporting it is an interesting adventure, one which I and my team, who work relentlessly behind the scenes, have worked out and handle unbelievably well. I have storehouses of equipment permanently stationed in Europe, the United States, and Japan. This means I can play on instruments that are familiar to me. I know how they "speak" and I save on wear and tear. I can have several instruments traveling around at once should concert dates be tightly scheduled. I have gone from country to country one day after the other with sometimes three technicians and three trucks all on separate routes! However, when I think of the wonderful time I experience as a touring solo percussionist, it is well and truly worth it.

There have been many "firsts" in my career, which has been unintentional, but since I am the first full-time solo percussionist, most of the things I do are "firsts." I gave the first solo percussion recital and concerto at the Henry Wood Promenade concerts in London; I was the first Western percussionist to give a concert tour of India; many of my concerto dates are the first time orchestras have put on percussion concertos; and I have premiered, thus far, around sixty new musical pieces. My whole career is, I suppose, like walking on a tightrope.

My musical role models are not only other percussionists but people like the late Glenn Gould, the famous Canadian pianist, who is the only musician I know whose ideas come vaguely close to my own thoughts, preferences, and perception of music. I also admire the late British cellist Jacqueline Du Pre, the young Russian pianist Evgeny Kissin, and the great Russian violist Yuri Bashmet. All of these people help me realize that I must forget that I am an instrumentalist and regard myself as a communicator who uses sound as a means of communication and emotion. I think this is where my habit of "playing by ear" or my fearlessness of the word "improvisation" is so helpful to me. I also believe music is medicine to us all and something we can all share.

In situations where I work with musicians who do not read music or have a totally different musical notation (such as in Indonesia) I realize that a sixth sense works in overdrive. My work with Björk, the fabulous Icelandic pop singer, proved to me that the willingness to be open-minded, to experiment, to imagine, and to work within the structure of the music proved to be of the utmost importance. Together we created, conducted, performed, and criticized our efforts, but all the time the childlike spontaneity of our work came through. This spontaneity is what I like to achieve in all my performances, whether playing with the New York Philharmonic, or Bartok's "Sonata for 2 Pianos and Percussion" with Sir Georg Solti and Murray Perahia, or in my private studio. I always visualize the audience and my performances in the privacy of my studio. Even my warm-up exercises are performed with an audience in my mind. In fact, visualization is one of the tools I use the most. Much of my practice is done away from my instruments, i.e., on planes and in airport terminals, so the ability to visualize is incredibly heightened. Some of my greatest performances have happened in my imagination while I walked through an airport.

The routine of my early days on the farm is a far cry from the variety of "a day in the life of Evelyn" now. I constantly travel throughout the world performing with the great orchestras and conductors, experiencing the wonderfully varied concert halls, cathedrals, theaters, palaces, and the fascinating cultures of the world, witnessing the power of music on whomever I meet. I count myself as very fortunate because I'm doing something I love. The joy of projecting this enthusiasm to others is immense. People assume that deafness means silence and therefore deaf people cannot enjoy or even comprehend music. The work of my favorite organization, the Beethoven Fund for Deaf Children, is a testament to the power of music to deaf youngsters. This fund was set up over ten years ago by a remarkable lady, Ann Rachlin, who runs courses for children called "Fun with Music." She narrates stories of the great classical music works. One day she asked herself, "Could deaf children experience what I'm giving my hearing children?" The answer was, of course, positive and now, among other things, the Beethoven Fund supplies quality instruments to schools for the deaf, as well as courses on how teachers for the deaf can utilize music as fun and therapy. In fact, the United Kingdom is now one of, if not the, leading country in the use of music with the deaf. This satisfaction of sharing one of life's essential ingredients is far beyond anything I can describe.

When I am asked what my plans are for the future; I reply simply to be happy in what I choose to do. If I am happy, other people will sense this. Of course, I experience ups and downs, as we all do, but those experiences give me strength and knowledge of myself.

Music is definitely my daily medicine.

Every instrumentalist walks with another shadow; a musician walks with his own shadow.

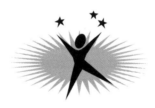

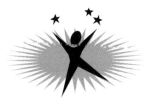

Conclusion

While researching this book, I became aware that all of the stories had common elements. All of the contributors saw a vision that they turned into a reality. No matter how many obstacles materialized, they kept focused on their goals. It amazes me that despite physical circumstances and challenges, each person featured in this compilation has made extraordinary contributions to their respective communities and to society as a whole. In addition to reaching their individual health and lifestyle goals, the contributors each touched hundreds of lives through their outreach efforts. They have all been honored with various prestigious awards from prominent public figures, colleges, and nonprofit organizations throughout the country. What can we learn from these journeys? All of the contributors, in their own special way, went through a process to successfully reach their goal.

All of them made a choice to take charge of the future. They defined what would bring them happiness. They decided what they wanted to accomplish in their lives and determined a goal in which they passionately believed. They made a commitment to keep focused on their goal. The long-term goal was broken down into smaller steps, and a timeframe was established for each step. Obstacles were viewed as challenges and overcome with flexibility, reflection, patience, and persistence. Gratification came from not only achieving their long-term objectives, but from conquering obstacles and accomplishing each step toward their goal.

Everyone can use this process to achieve individual dreams. When you believe that you have lost sight of your goals and feel lost, lonely, and confused, remember these individuals and their stories. By following their examples and determining what you want your purpose in life to be, you too can achieve happiness and satisfaction in your journey.